BOOK ENDORSEMENTS ~ PIONEERING VINYASA YOGA

David Swenson –

With this book Doug shares his knowledge through practical, down-to-earth instructions and inspiring, thoughtful stories. He guides the reader through an array of tools of self-discovery and encourages us each to tread our own path.

Take his book off of the shelf and dive into it. Swim through the life currents of Doug's nearly 50 years of living and breathing yoga and a healthy pathway toward self-discovery. You will be refreshed and discover new light shone on the steps of your own yogic/life journey!

David Swenson

Paul Grilley -

Doug Swenson is a bit of a legend. He has been mentioned with respect among many yogis I have known. I am honored to endorse his book.

Prana is the golden thread that ties together our physical, mental, and spiritual lives. Doug's book consistently follows this thread. It is rooted in asana practice but it branches from there into practices for the heart and mind.

I don't believe there will ever be one textbook of yoga, yoga is too vast. What we need are books that overlap in their outline of yoga but also share the unique ways each author has cultivated these practices. Doug's book is such a book. I hope it receives the wide readership that 50 years of dedicated practice can inspire.

Paul Grilley

Dharma Mittra –

Sharing spiritual knowledge is the highest type of charity. I believe that Doug Swenson and I have been sharing Yogic knowledge since the late 1960's or 70's, thus we have already passed through lots of experience and practice. So, this book is the result of practice and realizations.

Remember, only knowledge will dispel ignorance, and relieve pain and suffering. Nowadays, knowledge can easily be obtained: scriptures may be delivered overnight to your door. You can even find a guru online, but how to find the right one? Don't worry. When you are ready, this Divine book by Doug Swenson will appear.

~Dharma Mittra

Yogini Kaliji -

Reading Doug Swenson's words, the reader will feel the depth of his experience and his immersion in yoga. May his message on vegan lifestyle resonate with those whose life he touches. This book, expressed with such clarity, will be a source of inspiration for yogis now and for future generations.

Yogini Kaliji, the founder of TriYoga

Tao Porchon-Lynch -

Under the guidance of a teacher who truly activates each asana - the wonder of yoga radiates with true poetry in the meaning of life on this planet. Man becomes more aware of the eternal oneness of nature - and the inner reality with the breath of life radiates throughout the universe.

To you Douglas, who inspired the true Poetry of Yoga and these blessings of Nature to me and Bliss to all my students.

Thank you for the joy of yoga you have brought to us all - that opened the path for this gift of life. This to me is the very essence and beauty of the reality of yoga- The Music of the Soul.

Tao Porchon-Lynch

Jonny Kest –

Doug Swenson is a radical being! One who inspires you to go beyond your old limitations and break through your old conditioning to experience your full potential.

The word Yoga means relationship. Doug Swenson will share with you how to be in a relationship and come out successful!

Jonny Kest

Rodney Yee -

This new yoga offering from a tried and true yogi who has been resoundingly true to curiosity, service and love is a liberating inspiration. The stories are another testimony to the power and wonder of yoga and the practices presented are his authentic and tested pathways to presence and joy.

The cherry on top are the photographs that merge the majestic awe of nature and the brilliance of the human body in its exquisite forms.

Thank you Doug, Rodney Yee

David Life & Sharon Gannon -

Doug Swenson's passion for life and Yoga moves gracefully across the pages of Pioneering Vinyasa Yoga. The practices are interesting, challenging, and revealing, with lots of detail and photos. Doug's advice is rooted in ancient Yogic wisdom - illumined through the experiences of a modern yogi. Go with the Flow…

David Life, Jivamukti Yoga

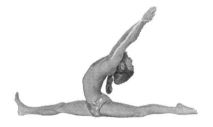

To know others is to find yourself ~ as moments become beads on the necklace of life.

PIONEERING VINYASA YOGA

THE ADVENTURE AND DAILY PRACTICE

Doug Swenson

Foreword by David Swenson

A SWENSON BOOK

A SWENSON BOOK

Published by Doug Swenson
1034 Emerald Bay Rd # 230
South Lake Tahoe, CA 96150
www.dougswenson.net

Ordering Information:
Quantity sales and special discounts are available on large volume purchases by corporations, associations, groups and individuals. For details, contact the author/publisher at the address above.

Orders by U.S. trade bookstores and wholesalers. Please contact the publisher:

Tel: (530) 573-8400; dougswen002@yahoo.com or visit www.dougswenson.net

Swenson trade paperback, first edition / February 2017

ISBN: 978-0-9984593-1-8

Library of Congress Cataloging-In-Publication data

Doug Swenson.
Pioneering Vinyasa Yoga: The Adventure and Daily Practice / Doug Swenson

ISBN: 978-0-9984593-1-8
1. Pioneering Vinyasa Yoga — 2017.

1 2 3 4 5 6   20 19 18 17

DEDICATION

I would like to dedicate this book to Patanjali, world renowned sage, yoga master, and author of the "Yoga Sutras." If it were not for the great effort and work, with all the practice and documentation of Yoga from Panjali, his students and those who came before him, very little information would be available for us today.

In addition, I feel it is important to dedicate this book to the ultimate best within each of you and hope this book will touch your heart and mind, inspiring your whole life and yoga practice, with awareness and compassion, intellect and creativity.

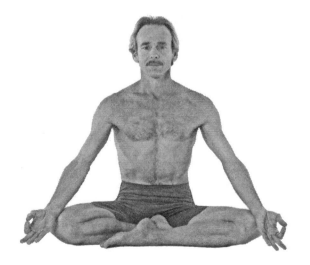

Santa Cruz, CA / 1975

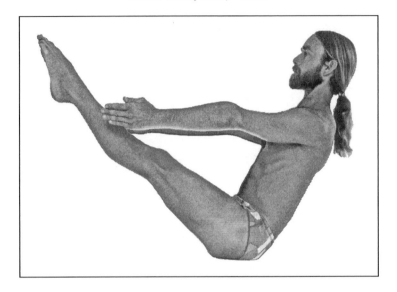

~ FORTY YEARS LATER ~

Lake Tahoe, CA / 2015

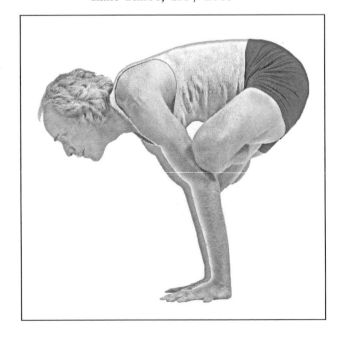

ACKNOWLEDGMENTS

I would like to express my overwhelming gratitude to these lovely souls

~ For their support, work and wonderful contributions ~

Blessings and Love, Doug Swenson

BACK STAGE CREW:

Foreword....................David Swenson (My amazing and talented little brother)

Photographers ....Rick Gunn, Addy Kaplan, Ram Photography

Publisher....................Doug Swenson / (Sadhana Yoga Chi)

Yoga Master.................Ernest Wood (Yoga Master / Sanskrit Scholar and Author)

Editors.......................Wendy White, Katarina Manos, Alex Keller & Douglas Dulac

Cover Design................Mladen Culic

YOGA MODELS:

Alex Keller, Almendra Garcia, Andrea Snyder, Ann Barros, Anna Ferguson, Christopher De Vilbiss, Colleen Saidman, Danny Paradise, David Life, David Swenson, Sri Dharma Mittra, Jan Thidarat Klinkularb, Jonny Kest, Joy Kunkanit, Kaya McAllister, Yogini Kaliji, Mark Stroud, Maya Cadengo, Nancy Gilgoff, Paul Grilley, Richardo Martin, Rodney Yee, Sara Turk, Seane Corn, Sharron Gannon, Shelley Washington, Suzie Grilley, Svetlana Panina, Tao Porchon Lynch and Yogi Hari.

ENDORSEMENTS:

David Life, David Swenson, Sri Dharma Mittra, Jonny Kest, Yogini Kaliji, Paul Grilley, Rodney Yee, Sharon Gannon and Tao Porchon-Lynch.

TASTE OF PHILOSOPHY

Where are you going?

Listen to your thoughts

As clouds

Should listen to the wind

Destiny Awaits

--------Doug Swenson

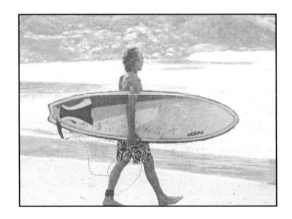

TABLE OF CONTENTS

PART I – SEEKING FOOD FOR THOUGHT

PART II – PIONEERING VINYASA YOGA / THE PRACTICE

PART III – FINDING BALANCE / HEALTH AND HAPPINESS

PART IV – LIVING THE PATH AND EVOLUTION OF YOGA

FOREWORD

By David Swenson

In life there are many circumstances, people and encounters that influence our character, personal choices, pathway and even our ultimate destiny. My older brother, Doug, has had an impact within all of these realms of my life and continues to inspire and encourage me in positive ways. Doug is and always has been a true trail-blazing visionary. He introduced me to Yoga in 1969 when very few people had any interest in it. In the early 1970's he wrote one of the first yoga books in the US, "Yoga Helps." By the mid-70's he wanted to share his love of nature, surfing, yoga and healthy living by making a yoga-surfing film titled, "Harmony Within." He inspired me to jump into the project as well. It took us 3 years to make and when completed we drove around the US and showed it in surf towns.

Doug has written many more books since "Yoga Helps," such as: "Mastering the Secrets of Yoga Flow," "The Diet that Loves you Most," and more. Doug steps lightly on this earth yet with deep compassion in his heart, sincerity in his actions and truth as his motivation. He is a poet, yogi, and surfer, a freethinker, role model, health crusader and big brother! His latest book, "Pioneering Vinyasa Yoga," is another expression of his deep insights into the realms of yoga and it's applications within all facets of life.

Doug shares his knowledge through practical, down-to-earth instructions and inspiring, thoughtful stories. He guides the reader through an array of tools of self-discovery and encourages us each to tread our own path. Take his book off of the shelf and dive into it. Swim through the life currents of Doug's nearly 50 years of living and breathing yoga and a healthy pathway toward self-discovery. You will be refreshed and inspired to discover new light shone on the steps of your own yogic/life journey!

With Greatest Love and Respect,

Doug's Little Brother, David

INTRODUCTION

The overall program of Pioneering Vinyasa Yoga is highly beneficial for all levels of students and teachers alike, including all ages, shapes, and sizes, from every walk of life. In this book, I present clear, updated, and easy-to-follow documentation for the practice of yoga, offered in a holistic and balanced format. By studying this book and my program, you will be inspired by the real life stories and adventures, gain an increased wisdom and awareness of the many aspects of yoga; and you will learn how to embrace yoga personally, so that its effects touch your whole life in a positive way. Everyone who makes a sincere effort to learn and practice this wonderful program will easily see how to introduce these concepts of yoga asana, diet and philosophy into their regular routine and by doing so will adopt a healthier and more conscious way of life.

I first started practicing yoga in 1963, at the age of 13. It has been over 50 years and I am still practicing today, at age 65. In the beginning, I was not really aware of exactly what yoga was and the vast benefits that yoga reflects on all aspects of life. No, at age thirteen, I was just being cool and trying to do a headstand. My exposure to yoga was purely by chance, or, more likely, fate. My parents did not practice yoga, and in 1963 yoga was not widely popular or fashionable in the U.S. — especially not in Houston, Texas!

My First Teacher - (Dr. Ernest Wood)

My parents belonged to a holistic and liberal church group "The Unitarian Fellowship." This church did not embrace any one tradition, or single concept. Instead, the group encouraged diversity and free thinking with respect for all others who held different visions. Destiny arrived as my father introduced me to one of the unique members of the church, Ernest Wood (Aug. 18, 1883 – Sept. 17, 1965), a true yoga master, theosophist, scholar and author of many books including "Concentration – An Approach to Meditation" (1949) and "The Pinnacle of Indian Thought" (1967).

The Seeds Were Planted

Ernest Wood and his teachings subconsciously became a part of my soul and although he passed away in 1965 when I was only 15, his message lived on within my mind. As time passed, I realized the priceless value of yoga and my practice gradually became very comfortable, and inspired, enabling me to acquire a greater sense of awareness. I realized my whole life was changing for the better. I was nicer to my parents; I could communicate better with all my friends, and found my job less stressful. My surfing improved greatly, I had an increasing desire to eat healthy food, and actually loved my yoga practice. My mind was feeling quite clear and I found myself wanting to learn more about life. My consciousness was expanding as I was drawn to climb a high plateau in the desert at sunset just to feel the energy of doing yoga on nature's stage.

Now, my yoga is a reflection of the ever-changing softness, strength and energy of nature. My connecting links *(Vinyasa),* flow in sync with the same energy, which governs the flow of the whole universe. I have learned to move with the life force of energy, rather than fighting against it. Yoga lifted the veil and I now see with more than my eyes.

Sadhana Vinyasa Yoga - is the name I have given to my style of yoga, which reflects a holistic philosophy. (*Sadhana*) means practice quest, or act of mastery, (*Vinyasa*) means to step or "place in a conscious manor," and (*Yoga*) means to "bring together" or unite. This quest for knowledge, moving forward in a conscious manor, comes together as a holistic program embracing a variety of essential concepts that are mindfully woven together as a garment of knowledge which will truly shed light on your yoga practice and touch your whole life in a positive way.

The most important and fundamental ingredient in any yoga practice and in all of life is prana, which means "vital life force." The awareness and utilization of Prana is the golden foundation in which Sadhana Vinyasa Yoga is built upon. Vital life force, or life force energy refers to the spark that separates living beings from non-living material. *Prana* is the core energy that connects all of us together and to the universe as a whole. In today's computerized, electronic and often hectic world, many of us have become very disconnected from prana. We tend to fight against the laws of nature rather than going with the flow. Sadhana Vinyasa Yoga represents a holistic yoga program! In this system you will discover the essence of how to revive a greater connection with vital life energy, being achieved with assistance from your yoga practice, healthy diet and lifestyle. In addition, you will easily see how you can find inner peace, strength, and relaxation within a beautiful flow of asana.

The vital life force, or prana, is not unique to humans. From the smallest single cell, to the infinite energy of a million galaxies and everything in between, the entire natural world is connected through energy. Each of us can learn to reap the benefits of living closer to this life force. By becoming one with prana, we can fuel our lives. It will drive us to reach our personal best no matter what we choose to do. Just as a fish separated from water cannot survive, and the beautiful colors of a flower cannot be seen without light; humans cannot reach their full potential if they separate themselves from the natural flow of universal energy.

Of course, all people achieve varying degrees of the essential partnership with prana. It is not simply an all-or-nothing concept. If you are alive, then you are embracing some degree of prana. However, most modern humans, due to poor lifestyle and improper diet, along with lack of exercise and scattered minds have lost out on a greater connection to prana and operate with very limited life force energy. But it can be done; everyone can enhance their life force energy, through the foundation of yoga asana practice and healthy diet, coupled with regular exercise and conscious living.

The effects can mean the difference between living an active, healthy life, or simply going through the motions and never really reaching your full potential. Those who reunite and cultivate enhanced life force energy can achieve conscious focus and a sense of inner peace, in addition to acquiring peak physical and mental performance at any age

Navigating the Structure of This Book

(The Sanskrit words are in italic, unless used repetitively or in common conversation).
In order for you to easily navigate the information and lessons of this book, I have divided this holistic presentation into four parts and fifteen easy-to-read chapters.

Part One:

"Seeking Food for Thought," this consists of three chapters to discover the essential foundation of Pioneering Vinyasa Yoga which will help you in your progress and enjoyment of the over-all program. In chapter one, you will be introduced to a true life story reflecting on how problems can be gifts in disguise, then in chapter two, you will come to understand the philosophy and background of yoga, presented in a easy to read and yet educational manor. In chapter three, you will learn many essential tips on how to build the foundation for a more progressive yoga practice, with many helpful suggestions and tools.

Part Two:

"Pioneering Vinyasa Yoga / The Practice," this consists of six chapters, beginning with chapter four, listing the instructions for a new approach to applying, mindful vinyasas and in chapter five you will find the details for practicing the yoga asana. Chapter's six, seven and eight offer yoga routines for different levels of practice. In chapter nine you will notice a very special chapter, for honoring Yoga teachers and daily *sadhana*. The overall message in Part Two embraces the concept of *vinyasa* (connecting links between yoga postures), with reference to awareness of energy in your whole life being compared to the energy of a river flowing to the sea.

Part Three:

"Finding Balance for Health and Happiness," this consists of four chapters to complement the balance of yoga practice. In chapter ten, you will learn wonderful techniques for meditation including helpful tips to assist in guiding you to success. Then in chapter eleven, you will find mindful and easy to read instructions for assisting with the science, art and practice of pranayama. In chapter twelve, you will discover the recipe for an enhanced and balanced yogic diet, which will improve every aspect of your life. In chapter thirteen, you will learn about body detox with *Yoga Kriyas* (internal cleansing), and restricted diet, to embrace a natural cleansing.

Part Four:

"Living the Path and Evolution of Yoga," this consists of two chapters which are, wonderful and priceless gifts. In chapter fourteen, you will enjoy four, fun, interesting, and adventurous stories of moments in time from my life and practice of yoga, which also presents the wider evolution of yoga in the western world. These stories touch on a time when yoga practice was not so popular or understood, and how it has evolved into the yoga practice of today. Chapter fifteen is the very last chapter, which aims to shed the light of philosophical awareness on your yoga practice and your whole life, by closing with a very inspirational, philosophical and poetic chapter reflecting on the journey and path of yoga, love and life.

If you can experience the treasured gifts in this book, as I have, you will quickly see how the benefits of this holistic Yoga program, are endless. And it all starts with planting a few positive seeds of thought, which soon grow into a vibrant and productive life.

Namaste, Doug

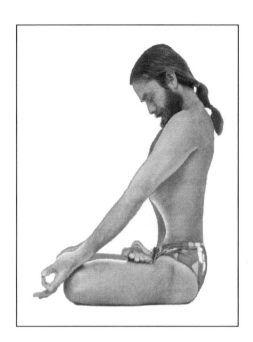

Photos – (Doug Swenson 1974)

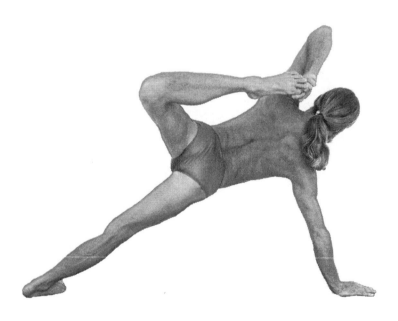

PART ONE

SEEKING

FOOD FOR THOUGHT

"There is no greater way to thank god for your sight
Than by helping others in the dark."

-----Helen Keller

CHAPTER 1

Hearing the Message
Unspoken

Have you ever had a dream, then awoke only to find it was not a dream at all, but a reality?

IN 1976, I traveled by car from my home base in Santa Cruz, Calif. back to Houston, Texas to visit my parents and teach a weekend, yoga workshop. I took about seven days to drive the 1,600 miles, stopping along the way to hike in Arizona, tube the rivers of West Texas, and practice yoga in some beautiful state parks with wildflowers flourishing in a symphony of colors.

Upon arriving at my parents' home, we spent the evening catching up on the latest family news. It seemed all was well with my parents. My mom, Violet, kept herself busy baking tasty pies and planting flowers in the garden while my father, Stanley, an attorney by trade, was spending his leisure time playing golf and watching sports.

My parents happily filled me in on my siblings' whereabouts and happenings. My little brother, David, was off in Encinitas, California practicing yoga, surfing and enjoying a blissful life, which made me feel proud since I was David's first yoga teacher and surfing inspiration. My big sister, Diana, was living not too far from Houston in the Woodlands, being a happy mom and becoming quite successful selling real estate, yet still pursuing her passion for dance.

The next morning, I drove off to teach the first day of my scheduled workshop on the other side of town. The workshop went very well, with about 20 students who all seemed to really enjoy my presentation of yoga. After class I took a few photos with the group and answered students' questions before I climbed into my trusty old Chevy Malibu and headed back to my parents' house.

As I drove down the road I could not help but feel gratitude and a sensation of being so very blessed — to be teaching something I loved, helping others and getting paid for it too. I was listening to a song on the radio by The Rolling Stones, singing the line, "You can't always get what you want, but if you try some time, you might just find - you get what you need." The song ended as I turned the radio off and next thing I knew, someone was talking to me in a calm yet concerned voice as they worked to pry open the door of my car. I vividly remember nice people asking me my name and what I did for a living, and I was more than happy to reply, excited that they wanted to hear about my way cool job as a yoga teacher.

One funny thing, they kept telling me everything would be all right, and I kept replying "Yes, of course everything will be all right. I am a yoga teacher — everything is always all right."

I thought I was dreaming, even as I found myself in an ambulance, alongside a nurse who kept asking if I had any pain.

"No, of course not," I replied. "I practice yoga and rarely, if ever, have any aches and pains." The dream continued as I woke up in a hospital bed with my right leg in traction, bandages on my head and intravenous tubes in my arms.

At that very moment I came to the terrifying realization that this was not dream, it was really happening. The nurse tried to calm me down as I frantically asked: "What happened? Where am I? What is going on?"

She called the doctor, and he explained I had been in a car wreck and broke my femur, had a serious concussion, and needed to calm down and relax. The doctor went on to inform me I was in a head-on collision with another car in which the driver and passenger were drunk. They sustained no serious injuries. I was not at fault, but I was devastated by my injuries and worried I would never be able to walk again, yet alone practice yoga asana and teach.

Little did I know that this horrible accident would later inspire my yoga creativity, and ultimately lead me to help many future students along a progressive path to a better life.

In the meantime, I searched for a reason why this happened to me. I believed in karma and contemplated as to what I did to deserve this rash punishment. Amidst the dark cloud of tragedy, my thoughts soon turned to how I could best achieve a quick recovery, get very healthy and leave the hospital as soon as possible.

In the days to come, after surgery to implant a steel rod inside my femur, I slowly regained my yogic survival instincts. Next came my will power and positive thoughts, one by one I turned down any and all non-essential drugs and medicines. Once this was achieved, I began trying to educate doctors and nurses on the true value of a healthy vegetarian diet, organics and green smoothies. But my effort was to no avail, as they kept bringing me meals of baby mush and processed sugary deserts.

I complained, but no one listened. On top of that, the doctor said I had to stay in the hospital for another 10 days to recover from my surgery!

"No F--ing way," I thought to myself. "I am a wilderness yogi, and I know damn well a caged bird cannot fly!"

During the hospital stay, my family took turns watching over me and the nurses dropped in on scheduled checks, yet in spite of my family's love and the nurse's support, I knew I had to search my mind for a way to get out sooner, I was feeling like a caged animal.

The next morning my family was gone for a bit, no nurses in sight, so I climbed up and over my bed railing. Myself and my newly-implanted femur rod crawled along the floor and over to the wall. I had to rest and catch my breath for about 10 minutes! I was not my normal self, which seemed to me all the more reason to proceed with my plan, which was to do a headstand against the wall, without my hospital gown — only my birthday suit and yoga mentality. I asked my roommate to wait until I was inverted, then ring the bell for emergency assistance. He smiled, with a sparkle in his eyes and agreed!!!

OK. Up we go. I was feeling quite dizzy and fragile, but managed the headstand. My roommate laughed, the buzzer rang and a few seconds later, in rushed three nurses.

"Oh my God," the head nurse exclaimed. "What the heck do you think you are doing? You need bed rest." Yet behind the words, she had a nice smile!

She scurried me back into my gown and my hospital gurney, being very professional and yet intrigued with a playful and curious mind. But the plan worked! The very next day, my doctor signed my release papers and I got to go home, in care of my family — but not before turning down my prescription for pain pills. I was convinced that yoga breathing, meditation, and my positive thoughts were all I needed.

Being at my parents' house was both a blessing and a curse. They were kind, caring souls, but I greatly missed my independence, like-minded yoga mates, and nature. The next day I quietly escaped very early and slipped out the back door with my crutches. I made my way down to the end of the street where a springtime flower meadow waited patiently for my arrival.

I sat down within the symphony of flowers and bathed in the bliss of sunlight. Like a plant that had gone too long without water, I drank in my surroundings, quickly reviving my spirit and prana. Then, I noticed something very cool. Four or five butterflies floated in the afternoon breeze and to my surprise, landed right on my broken leg. Within seconds I was hypnotized by this amazing phenomena. Suddenly, like a light in the darkness an incredible feeling came over me, and I started to cry uncontrollably. My heart was full of tremendous joy and unconditional love.

At that moment I heard an unspoken message as if it were being said out loud and clear: *"From tremendous pain and suffering can arrive something beautiful, magical and healing, something full of love."*

At that moment I knew what I had to do. I was destined to write a book on yoga. I wanted to help people overcome stress and discomfort. I wanted to bring sunny springtime meadows into the darkness of lost hearts. I wanted to inspire healing and share what I had come to truly believe with all my heart and soul: the fact that yoga truly helps.

I followed my destiny, and used my time off to pioneer one of the first yoga books written in the U.S. It was rightfully titled "Yoga Helps." Ironically, about six months later I received an insurance settlement for $30,000. Although my parents wanted me to buy a house and marry the girl next door, I used the money to self-publish my first yoga book in 1978.

In this spiral bound book, with a photo of myself on the cover sporting long hair and a full beard, sitting in lotus in my beloved field of wildflowers, I shared photos, illustrations and instructions for yoga asana, Sun Salutations and pranyama, as well as inspirational thoughts.

"Yoga Helps" was an easy to digest, simplistic, and self-published yoga practice book. The melody of the book was a gentle approach to a balanced practice. My brother David agreed to pose for some photos in the book and impart some helpful advice, along with our very cool neighbor and one of our first students Laurie. "Yoga Helps" was also one of the first yoga books published in the U.S. to introduce the concept of vinyasa yoga and **the first book in the U.S.** to dedicate one chapter to the practice of what we then called "The Series" which is now known as **"Ashtanga Yoga."**

At the time and place I wrote this book, there were very few yoga studios, only a handful of yoga styles and definitely no yoga mats, or fashionable props in Walmart! My brother David and I stood up proud and practiced yoga when yoga was not cool and often had very challenging residual effects.

Like one fun day, when all the neighbors collectively called the police because there were two suspicious young men doing strange things in the park, behind the trees. And another time when a younger boy shot at us with his BB gun as we were practicing yoga. Then the slow passive resistance of well-meaning citizens with visions of darkness and evil energy taking over yoga minds and spilling beyond into the surrounding neighborhood.

Today, "seeing the world through another's eyes," all these accounts now seem perfectly reasonable to me. Because at the time Yoga was not understood, it was different and not fashionable, so justified caution and fear embraced the hearts and minds of those who had an unexpected (encounter of the fourth kind).

No this is not a typo!!! I said, "Encounter of the Fourth Kind," not a UFO but a UFY, you know, "Unidentified Flying Yogi."

Now out of print, but never out of mind, the ripples in time from this endeavor have touched many. I have been told by many people over the years, on how my book "Yoga Helps" exposed them to yoga for the first time, and that it helped them cultivate practice at a time when yoga was less accessible in this country, let alone fashionable or cool. My book also planted seeds for future authors, including my own brother, David, who went on to publish the amazing book "Ashtanaga Yoga the Practice," which has touched hearts and minds around the world with positive light and inspired a whole new culture and yoga following.

Since then I have written 3 books on yoga, one of enhanced diet, in addition to teaching yoga workshops around the world. I have always found time for my yoga and continue to practice virtually every day. Through all this, my underlying conviction hasn't changed: "Yoga helps, it really does!!!"

Communication is the highest note in spirituality
You play your note and they play theirs
And yet - there is no music...

There is no music...
Until each individual note
Becomes one

As a beautiful symphony is born
Darkness turns to light
And flowers bloom in winter

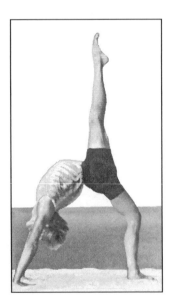

—————

CHAPTER 2

Viewing Evolution
The Philosophy of Yoga

Become a humble beginner and empty your cup
Fill your heart with awareness
Creating a universe ~ of Body Mind and Soul

Not so long ago, an aspiring *yogi* or *yogini,* such as you, would have had to travel great distances over frozen mountains and across blazing desserts to find a worthy teacher. Upon finding this teacher, you would then be subjected to sleeping in the snow, fasting for 30 days, practicing your yoga in a nasty room full of poisonous snakes, or enduring many other physical and mental tests. Of course this is just a colorful, inspired metaphor and an extreme example, but in reality, students would usually be asked to endure dedication and trials to prove they were worthy of studying yoga in a serious way. Your choices of yoga teachers also would have been greatly limited: as compared to present day popularity of practicing and teaching yoga.

Now that yoga practice seems to have reached just about every country of the world, the availability and variety of teachers has grown as well. The good news is you no longer have to climb a tall peak or hike over scorching sands of a desert to find a great teacher, and there are a wide variety of yoga styles to choose from.

I have great respect and appreciation for all styles of yoga and for those who have endeavored to teach the various systems of yoga. Because of the efforts of the many individuals who practice and teach yoga, this science and healing art has touched our society in a very positive and nurturing way.

One of the most acknowledged and respected original texts on yoga, "The Yoga Sutras" of Pantajali, categorized yoga as an eight-limb path. The trunk and limbs that connected this eight-fold path represent the one common ground that all yoga teachings embrace. All styles of yoga are structured to improve quality of life, and awareness through a series of physical and mental disciplines. Patanjali further sub-classified yoga into smaller categories or branches. Each of the separate branches sprouted from the eight larger limbs as you will see in the following explanation.

THE EIGHT LIMBS OF YOGA

(As outlined in the "Yoga Sutras" of Patanjali)

(1) *Yama* – Abstinences:

(a) Ahimsa – Embrace peace and non-violence.

(b) Satya – Be truthful and honest in all ways.

(c) Asteya – Refrain from stealing and cheating.

(d) Brahmacharya – Maintain integrity of intimate relationships.

(e) Aparigraha – Refrain from hoarding, be free from the bonds of materialism.

(2) *Niyama* – Observances:

(a) *Saucha* – Strive for purity in body, mind and spirit.

(b) Santosa – Embrace contentment within simplicity, and feel tranquility.

(c) *Tapas* – Endure work and hardship in exchange for an improved body and mind.

(d) *Svadhyaya* – Embrace self-study and always see yourself as a student.

(e) *Isvara* – Be humble in the presence of the Supreme Being, or vital life force energy.

(3) *Asana* – Postures:

The practice of sacred yoga postures for physical and mental health.

(4) *Pranayama* – Breathing:

The science, art, and practice of enhanced breathing techniques.

(5) *Pratyahara* – Sense Withdrawal:

Is withdrawal of the senses in order to gaze inward and maintain clear focus.

(6) *Dharana* – Concentration:

This implies to focusing your entire energy on one particular area of thought.

(7) *Dhyana* – Meditation:

Is Gaining control over your mind with sustained, effortless, and relaxed intellect.

(8) *Samadhi* – Self Realization:

To reach enlightenment, shed the ego, and become one with the universe.

Basic Philosophy and Background of Yoga

The basic philosophy of yoga is centered on creating balance and awareness between your physical, mental, and spiritual self. This balance can be achieved through disciplines of physical and mental exercises, breathing techniques, deep relaxation, and following a pure diet. The end result is a connection with the natural flow of energy in the universe.

Wise sages and *gurus* believed the answers to the questions on how humans could live a healthier and more productive life were found in the hands of Mother Nature. From studying different forms of life, these wise sages came to the conclusion that there was a sacred balance of strength and softness within all creatures and within nature itself. In time, their teachings evolved into a practical system that was handed down from teacher to student over thousands of years. The connection of an improved diet, along with techniques of fasting, the evolution of yoga postures and mental training techniques, formed the system that we now refer to as *yoga*. This system created a positive direction for all humans to follow in order to greatly enhance their physical, mental, and spiritual health.

Hatha Yoga Philosophy

Hatha yoga refers to the practice and mastery of physical yoga postures, and it is the base discipline of many yoga styles today. Individual postures are called *asanas*, which translates as "position comfortably held," or "seat." When done correctly, each *asana* creates a very powerful source of vital life force energy and has many anatomical benefits.

The most popular and widely used techniques of yoga practice today are really a combination of the traditional branches of *Hatha*, *Raja*, and *Prana* yoga. *Hatha* basically increases your physical health through "practicing yoga postures" while *Raja* is "mastery of the mind" and *Prana* is "awareness of breath coupled with vital life energy." The melding of the three categories promotes balanced physical and mental health, and a union between *yin* and *yang*, or feminine and masculine energies. The goal of *Hatha* yoga combined with *Raja* and *Prana* yoga is to achieve a body of perfect health and strength, to inspire a relaxed mind, yet aware and perceptive, this combined with the ability to embrace peace and harmony in your heart leading to an unbridled vision of all life.

Evaluating Your Energy Source

As you have learned, the practice of yoga connects you with the natural flow of energy throughout the universe. Yoga creates an enormous amount of positive energy. You can choose to store your *prana* on the shelf and let it sit there to collect cobwebs, or put this wonderful and magical gift to work. Sadhana Vinyasa Yoga is especially designed to help you access your full energetic potential, through a holistic approach. The realization of what you have is the first step along the path to using this energy to assist you throughout every aspect of life.

Yoga philosophy is all about awareness and tapping into your full potential, utilizing your body, mind, and spirit in full bloom, unrestricted from the distractions of everyday society. If you can use only a minor portion of this energy created from your yoga practice in your daily life, many good things will happen.

PIONEERING VINYASA YOGA (The Philosophy)
~ Seven Key Parts of a Holistic Practice ~

(1) Integrity of Daily Living
Embrace a positive outlook and inspire non-violence ~
Being truthful, humble and respectful with a loving heart.

(2) Asana Practice
Create a holistic balance between (hard & soft) asana practice ~
Reflecting a mindful and progressive vinyasa.

(3) Meditation and Spirituality

Quiet your mind and inspire your soul with awareness ~

As you become the light in darkness for others.

(4) Cross Training

Occasionally practice other styles of Yoga for a broader vision ~

Embrace cross-training outdoors with conscious appreciation of your surroundings.

(5) Healthy Diet

Educate yourself, striving to improve and adopt better habits ~

Respect your body as your temple, knowing you deserve healthy food

Discovering that food becomes thought and thought motivates action!

(6) Karma Yoga

Show gratitude and respect for ecology and all life ~

Promote random acts of kindness, as priceless gifts in the stream of life.

(7) Sense of Humor

Teach laughter as the best medicine ~

Mindfully weave happiness with intellect, inspiring souls to bloom.

This style of Sadhana Vinyasa Yoga is very balanced and complete in itself, however I truly believe the essence of yoga should not be confined to an unbending, very structured and packaged system. Learn what you can, then add this to the new and different knowledge you will discover outside the confines of the box.

That being said, I encourage you to use my system as your base, yet on occasion open the box and go out to study and practice some of the other wonderful systems of yoga, along with any other progressive mind body philosophies and techniques. In doing so, you will return to Sadhana Vinyasa Yoga with fresh perspective and enhanced wisdom.

All great philosophies need open minded students, to embrace the light and inspire growth as flowers of inspiration blossom into enhanced wisdom.

Yoga practice opens the door
Thus prana may find you

~ ~ ~

In the garden of this life
Where colorful thoughts bloom
And peace prevails

~ THE 16 BRANCHES OF YOGA ~

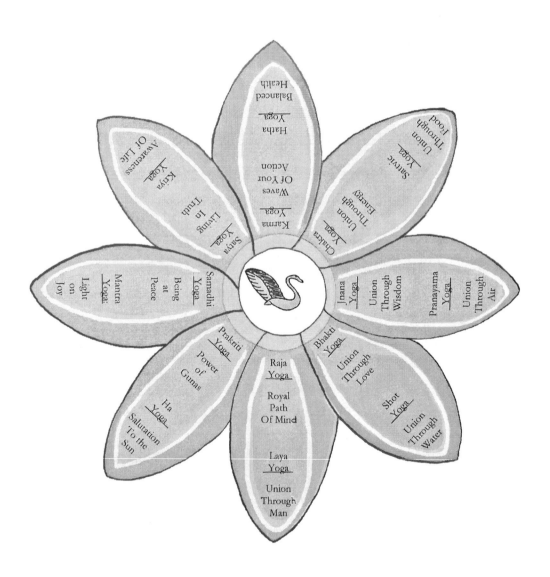

CHAPTER 3

Building the Foundation
For Practice

The mindful gardener - will grow deep roots
Before climbing the tree

In this chapter, you will discover a method of choosing the yoga asana practice best suited for your personal needs, along with a checklist to evaluate the approach designed for you. Next, you will find some helpful suggestions and a list of yoga tools to assist you in practice, as well as a basic outline for yoga breathing. Lastly, I will describe six qualities of yoga asana, which will give you a better understanding of how, why, and when to practice yoga asana.

Yoga is a very individualized practice. Unlike competitive activities where you strive to become the single winner, in yoga, everyone is a winner. With yoga practice, it is a good idea to find a main base practice, style and teacher which feels right for you - but then occasionally learn from other teachers and styles. Over time, your interest may change to something completely different as you evolve with your practice and life. This evolution of practice, along with adding the other elements of Sadhana Vinyasa Yoga (meditation, diet, cross-training, and philosophy) will soon lead you to the ultimate yoga experience!

I often refer to physically demanding yoga practice as Hard Flow and the less physically demanding as Soft Flow. Through the practice of Sadhana Vinyasa Yoga you choose your own level of challenge, remembering you always have control over your practice. If you want to work hard and really build your muscles, try a strenuous, (Hard) yoga routine. If you want to enjoy a less challenging practice, try an easy (Soft) practice. You can even structure a little of both into one routine. You may also vary the pace, by speeding up or slowing down your vinyasa flow, which can create different results depending on your motives.

With this holistic concept in mind, there are certain choices you need to make, as well as key techniques that need to be studied. Your first decision is the level of intensity you would like to have in your practice. Control over the amount of physical work within your yoga routine is achieved through four variables: your choice of yoga postures, how you practice your postures, the length of time you hold the postures, and your choice of vinyasa. Plus, there is always a place for the use of yoga tools and props, which can and do help in all levels of practice.

LEVELS OF INTENSITY / BALANCING THE FOUR VARIABLES

Envision a peaceful river winding through the countryside. As gentle as this river seems, you know that it is strong enough to carve a path through solid rock. What you are observing is the marriage between softness and strength. Maybe you really enjoy a slower pace, with less intensity, or a faster pace with more intensity while still challenging your body and building stamina, Sadhana Vinyasa Yoga can accommodate both. The key, again, is in how you choose your postures, how long you hold the poses and which type of vinyasa you choose.

1) Choice of Yoga Postures

The yoga postures themselves have a great deal to do with the level of challenge in your practice. Some postures are very easy to embrace without having to defy gravity or balance on your arms. On the other hand, if you want a greater physical challenge you need to do something other than lie flat on your back in the Corpse Pose in order to get your internal turbo boost charged.

You may choose a specific routine and stick to it over time, but elect to try alternative posture variations as listed in Chapter Five to find an asana intensity which suits your present level.

Or you may vary your entire practice routine from day to day, or week to week, choosing the one which best suits your needs at any given time. In this book, I have structured each routine with alternatives and suggestions for those who want to build a slightly different sequence.

2) Yoga Posture Variations

The manner in which you practice your yoga postures also has an impact on the level of physical challenge in your routine. For example, if you are practicing a very challenging standing posture like Warrior II, you can make it even more challenging by sinking deeper into your lunge. Or, you can make the posture less challenging by backing off a bit, using props and conserving your energy for another pose. The most difficult path is not necessarily the best, the intelligent yoga students and teachers will vary their practice routines and intensity for a more successful outcome. Try to always be aware of your ego in yoga practice, there are times when your ego will render you blind of common sense and mindful judgement.

3) Length of Asana Holds

The length of time you choose to stay in an individual yoga posture can also affect the challenge level and intensity. Even a non-strenuous posture such as Tree Pose can be very demanding if you hold it for a much longer time. On the other hand, if you are practicing a difficult arm balance like Crane Pose and only hold the posture for a few seconds, then you have not created much of a challenge. I suggest you build up gradually, and periodically vary the length of time you hold your yoga asanas.

One idea is to pick one week every few months and practice fewer postures in your daily routine, but hold each asana for a longer duration. In this manner your practice length remains the same overall, only you stay in your postures longer. After the week of longer holds you can return to your normal routine. This is a safe and effective way to build endurance and stamina. Of course, you could go the opposite way and make the special week easier by doing yin or restorative yoga. Please refer to the (Chapters 6 – 8) for practice routines to fit your needs.

4) Choice of Vinyasa

Your choice of vinyasa and the speed, or pace, of your vinyasa can quite dramatically affect your level of physical challenge. In Chapter Four, I provide you several choices between more and less challenging flows to connect your postures together. The more challenging vinyasa will work your muscles to a much greater degree as you resist your body weight against gravity. In some cases, the more challenging vinyasa is a more involved movement. For example, you may move from lying on the floor, up to standing, and back to the floor again, all as one vinyasa. In the less challenging vinyasa, the muscle resistance factor is much lower, and in some cases the movements are less involved and very subtle, like lifting your arms up over your head and back down again. In the chapter on vinyasa, I also suggest using different pacing for varied outcomes.

HOW TO CREATE A CHALLENGING PRACTICE - (Four Helpful Tips)

When yoga was first introduced to the Western world, the idea of achieving a good physical workout through yoga practice was literally unheard of. However, since the early '70s, with the introduction of Ashtanga Yoga, and then other styles which have since emerged introducing a very physical and challenging workout (hard flow) yoga is now at your fingertips. If you are looking to increase your muscle challenge and cardiovascular capabilities as well, Sadhana Vinyasa Yoga can offer this type of Hard Flow workout.

1. Getting a Cardio Workout with Yoga

Sadhana Vinyasa Yoga can fulfill a challenging cardio workout, similar to Power Yoga and Ashtanga Yoga, especially if you choose a more challenging routine to practice. Yet in addition, I always advise my students to seek cardio outside of yoga practice. Cardio capabilities vary from one individual to the next. Getting your heart rate up to at least 70 percent of its maximum power and sustaining this for at least 15 minutes is the true measure of what is considered to be a beneficial cardio activity. If you are a marathon runner, you will have to work harder to get to your optimal aerobic workout level than someone who is out of shape.

The good thing is you can reach the minimum requirements for an aerobic workout within Sadhana Vinyasa Yoga, but to do this you have to challenge yourself. Resting in a Forward Bend will not get you where you want to go. However, remember that you don't have to race through your routine in order to get more of an aerobic workout in yoga. You can move slowly and still strengthen your heart and lungs. Once again, I believe it is best to seek additional cardio/aerobic exercising in your daily life, outside of yoga.

2. Discovering Muscle Resistance Through Yoga

If you are seeking muscle resistance, you can find quite a lot within Sadhana Vinyasa Yoga, although it is best to look at your practice and make sure you are doing weight-bearing exercises for all areas of the body. I suggest you also add alternative weight-bearing exercises outside of yoga, to balance your overall lifestyle. There are several factors which influence the strength building aspects of your yoga practice. In yoga, anaerobic exercise is achieved in several ways: through use of your own body weight, holding yoga postures, moving from one position to another, partner adjustment work, and isometric exercise.

3. Blending Cardio and Muscle Resistance

Each yoga asana or vinyasa ranges within a spectrum of intensity. For example, a Seated Forward Bend takes very little strength to complete, while a Handstand is very physically demanding on the upper body. In the Seated Forward Bend, you are getting very little anaerobic exercise, mostly just stretching the back side of your body. On the other hand, in the Handstand you are pushing your own body weight up over your head, much like weight lifting. You can choose the amount of strenuous postures to work into your routine, thereby controlling the duration of anaerobic exercise within your yoga practice.

4. Progress with Awareness

As in any anaerobic activity, gradually work up to more challenging, strength-building yoga routines. As a newcomer to yoga the best thing to do is take it easy, try out a beginner level routine, and see how you feel. Then gradually increase your challenge and you will find that you enjoy your yoga practice much more.

HOW TO CREATE A SOFT PRACTICE - (Three Helpful Tips)

Yoga practice is about choices and you can certainly embrace a softer, and less challenging practice. In this section I have listed three suggestions to assist in a softer yoga practice.

1. Energy Management

There are two diametrically different results from experiencing a yoga practice: you can either feel depleted of energy and end up being tired afterward, or you can enhance your energy and find yourself refreshed afterwards. In a softer practice, you should embrace a relaxed and non-rushed attitude, instead of challenging your asanas and striving to conquer them, try to make friends with your yoga poses and find comfort in their presence. In this manor you will find it works especially well with those who are seeking the easy or soft form practice.

If you move too fast without awareness and fail to focus on your deep breathing, you waste a lot of strength unnecessarily and will ultimately be losing your potential energy, depleting strength and mental clarity. The solution is found within learning to be aware in your practice, being in touch with your heart and mind as you really feel the actions being cultivated.

2. Varying the Pace

Something as simple, as modifying your pace of movement in the yoga vinyasa can have a large impact on the end result. Move slower to cool your body, quiet your mind, and lengthen your breathing flow, instilling a sense of inner calm, to greatly enhance a softer practice

3. Choosing Asanas Wisely

The yoga postures themselves have a great deal to do with the level of challenge in your practice. Some postures are very easy to practice, while others are very strenuous. This all depends on your motives and needs, choose your asana wisely. **For the softer practice stay away from arm balances, move at a slower pace and use less strenuous vinyasa**. If you want a soft practice, avoid the muscle resistance based vinyasa with challenging poses.

Strive to rotate your practice, creating a delicate balance of strength and softness.

THREE INTERNAL TOOLS / FOR SUCCESSFUL PRACTICE

1. Develop Mind Flow

Very few of us function with our body and mind in unison. If you can totally connect your thoughts with your actions, the results are quite amazing. In sports, dance, martial arts, or leisure activities, a mind-body connection can mean the difference between falling on your face or smoothly gliding with grace and elegance.

One of the main goals of yoga is the unification of mind-body action. You have to master your mind before you can master your body. Whether you choose to follow a Hard or Soft Flow workout, you also need to develop your yoga practice from within. Your own beautifully flowing, yet powerfully physical yoga practice mirrors your beautiful yet powerful mind and inward energy. During Sadhana Vinyasa Yoga, we strive to embrace the mind-body connection at all times, yet with relaxed focus and inner calm. Your thoughts are in the moment, not scattered, or thinking of other worldly issues. Only when mind and body are working together can true harmony and grace be achieved.

2. Drishti: Focus on the Internal Gaze

In some yoga styles, much emphasis is placed on the way you direct and hold your gaze during practice. "Fixed focal points" are assigned for each posture, and are called *drishti*. The word *drishti* means both "looking out" and "looking in."

The purpose of the *drishti* is not to get you looking at a particular place or part of your body; it's actually an exercise to help you turn your gaze inward, so that you can place your attention on your breathing, posture alignment and *bandhas* "internal locks." Gazing inward is considered to be a form of sense withdrawal, and the drishti is a tool to help you in this part of yoga practice. When you use the drishti you are more focused on your internal yoga, and less apt to be distracted by external things. This gaze has an impact on your physical and mental state during each posture, and your ability to remain focused and energized.

In Pioneering Vinyasa Yoga, students are taught to gaze into a posture's "energy line." This means to focus the drishti in the direction of your stretch in any given posture and then turn your focus inward. Students are also encouraged to focus on the line of least resistance, which can be an individualized aspect. For example, if you are very flexible and practicing a Seated Forward Bend, gazing at your toes will create tension in your neck. In this case you would lower your vision toward your legs. On the other hand, a less flexible person will find least resistance by gazing at their toes. Personally, I prefer not to be too strict with the drishti, and have found through experience the aspect of gazing in the direction of the stretch and the individualized approach of gazing along the lines of least resistance to be most useful.

3. **Bandhas: Gateways of Internal Power**

The first natural tool your mind can make use of during yoga practice is the *bandha*, or "energy lock." You engage a bandha through the concentrated effort of contracting certain muscles within your body. These contractions, or locks, direct the flow of the prana energy you create during yoga practice, while helping to create stability and inward strength. Bandhas give your mind and your entire body an energy lift during your vinyasas. They also offer you added control during your asanas, as well as tone up your stomach and internal organs. By engaging your bandhas, you maintain greater control and focus over your body's actions, which leads to the knowledge that you can control and focus your mind as well. When practicing bandhas, be subtle and gentle.

Bandhas are actually muscle locks or pressure points within your body. **Each of the three primary bandhas used in this system has its own name and is explained below.**

To get the most out of your practice, you should engage your *mula* and *uddiyana bandhas* each time you hold a yoga posture, then release the bandhas as you leave a posture. Re-engage the bandhas during your vinyasa linking movements. They will give you extra strength when the vinyasa involves lifting your body weight.

THE THREE BANDHAS

1. Mula Bandha:

Mula Bandha is also known as the "root lock", and is located in the perineal muscles between your genitals and anus. To engage these muscles, moderately lift the pelvic floor during the yoga asana. Try to be relaxed. Don't strain. Then, release your *mula bandha* when you are ready to exit the asana. In yoga practice, if you are practicing a muscle resistance vinyasa, you may re-engage *mula bandha* to create lift and defy gravity for a fluid vinyasa.

2. Uddiyana Bandha:

The name *Uddiyana* translates as "flying up." This bandha is located about three fingers below your navel. To engage this *bandha*, focus on your lower abdominal muscles as you lift and contract them slightly, which then draws up your diaphragm. During asana practice, *uddiyana bandha* is usually used in conjunction with *mula bandha*. Together, they give you strength and stability, while firming your abdominal muscles and helping you embrace greater prana energy.

3. Jalandhara Bandha:

The *jalandhara bandha* is also called the "chin lock." You engage this *bandha* by stretching the back of the neck as you lower your chin into the notch in your breastbone. You engage this *bandha* naturally in a few poses like Shoulder Stand and Staff, yet more frequently in some pranayama breathing exercises. You will not use *jalandhara bandha* nearly as often as you use the *mula bandha* or the *uddiyana bandha*. Anatomically, some people will not be able to achieve full jalandhara bandha- no worries, just tilt your chin toward your chest.

Being Mindful of the Moment

You can accomplish a lot more in your life, and your yoga practice, by being present in the moment, totally aware of all that is going on around you, in control and at peace. If you always think of how things will get better later, or how you will relax and do what you want later on, the time may never arrive. In yoga practice you should enjoy special and sacred moments as precious gifts. Be in the moment; experience the struggle as much as the blissful relaxation. Live your life for today.

"Life is what happens ~ when you are busy making other plans" --- **John Lennon**

Your mind is a reflection of your physical actions; therefore, changes in your body also affect your emotional state. Once you embrace the essence of yoga, you will experience a more focused mind and feel a direct connection with the natural flow of energy. As you notice more physical energy, you will also notice an increase in mental energy, whether you are reading books, organizing your thoughts, working, or just relaxing with a friend or loved one. You will develop a sense of well-being, greater self-confidence, and find yourself in tune with positive thoughts. Everyone will love to be around you as you find it easier to communicate and touch the hearts of others.

YOGA BREATHING MADE SIMPLE

The Sanskrit word *pranayama* refers to the "science and practice of breath control." It is a combination of two important terms, *prana*, meaning "vital life force," and a*yama*, which means "to extend." Prana represents all the elements of life: earth, air, fire, water, and ether. Yoga practice helps you extract these elements from nature through controlled breathing, which replenishes pranic energy. Taking this concept one step further, many great yoga masters have expressed the idea that air is a food. They believe that if you cleanse the body of toxins and live in a clean, fresh environment, then air can serve as a supplemental nutritional source. The best, most highly-charged air is available near mountains, waterfalls, and oceans — all areas abundant with negatively-charged ions. I can tell you from experience that when I practice yoga in places with a good supply of negatively-charged ions it is incredibly powerful.

In our daily lives, most of us tend to take very shallow breaths. Over time this incomplete breathing can reduce our overall health and vitality. Yoga breathing is quite different from regular breathing. By consciously making an effort to maintain correct breathing, we are rewarded with more energy, less stress, and better mental focus. With each breath, you will better oxygenate your blood and muscles, and supply fresh oxygen to your brain. You will be expanding your lungs, greatly increasing their capacity and ability to fuel your body. What's more, the slow and deep breathing rhythm in Sadhana Vinyasa Yoga builds energy while at the same time generating a calm, yet focused mind during both Hard and Soft Flow practice, as well as in your everyday life.

THREE DISTINCT QUALITIES OF YOGA BREATHING:

1. **The complete breath:** For each breath you take, completely fill your lungs with air on inhalation (*puraka*) and completely empty your lungs on exhalation (*rechaka*).

2. **Slow deep breathing:** In Sadhana Vinyasa Yoga, your breathing is slow, steady, deep, and rhythmic. This controlled breathing enables you to pull more oxygen into your lungs, leaving you feeling refreshed and invigorated after practice. It also creates a calm and relaxed mind.

3. **Sound breathing:** *Ujjayi,* or "victorious breath," involves inhaling and exhaling air through your nose. As you breathe in and out through your nose, you create a soft, hissing sound on the back of your throat. This tranquil, meditative sound helps to regulate the volume and pace of the air you breathe. Your slow, deep, calculated breathing pattern enhances energy, calms the body and mind, and enables you to center your thoughts on your practice.

THE SIX QUALITIES OF YOGA ASANA

After 40 years of researching the practice of yoga asana, I have created a holistic outline, or checklist, in order to help you see in which areas you may be restricted, or could be enhanced. There are some postures that will never be your cup of tea while others will come easy for you. In poses that are difficult, simply modify and use awareness. Here are six factors that can affect your ability to achieve asana:

1. **Flexibility:** The flexibility of your muscles, ligaments and joints, are determined in part by genetics and plays a big role in dictating which yoga asanas you find easy or hard.
2. **Strength:** Many poses involve muscle strength, but we really need to find a true balance between strength and flexibility embracing a more holistic practice.
3. **Balance:** Having good balance is an advantage in many yoga asanas, however we need to combine balance with the other yoga asana qualities to optimize our practice.
4. **Technique:** Technique is the base foundation of your yoga asana. Think like an architect as you mindfully build your poses, success will become you.
5. **Self-confidence:** Self-confidence will help in many aspects of yoga practice, but too little will hold you back and too much self-confidence can result in injury.
6. **Body Type:** We are each completely unique, discovering certain yoga asana that will fit very well with our inherited body type, and others that will not. Some poses we assume naturally and some take work and patience. Still, in others postures, we are only able to partially achieve, despite even our persistent effort.

Previous and present injuries can also be an issue in practicing yoga asana
~ Be mindful and always practice with awareness ~

DOUG SWENSON / PHOTO GALLERY (1972 – 2016)

Year / 1972

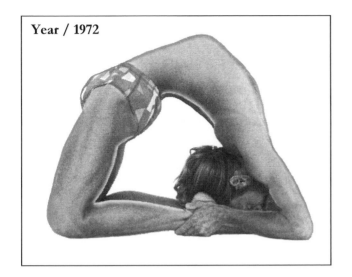

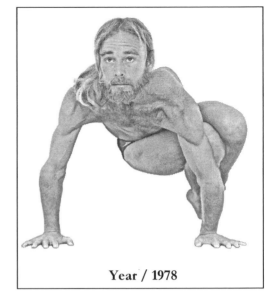

Year / 1978

Year / 2016

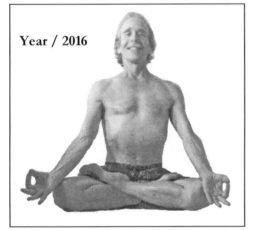

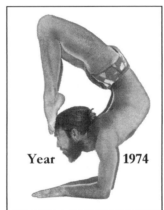

Year   1974

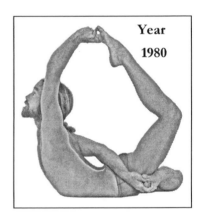

Year
1980

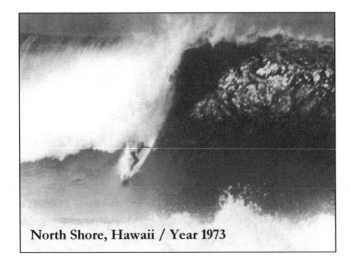

North Shore, Hawaii / Year 1973

Year / 2010

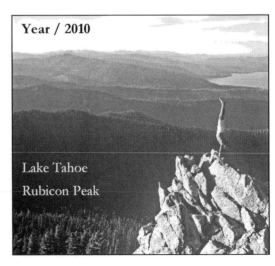

Lake Tahoe
Rubicon Peak

PART TWO

PIONEERING VINYASA YOGA

THE PRACTICE

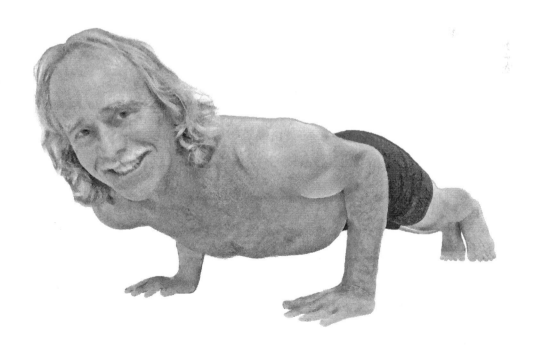

CHAPTER 4

Studying Vinyasa
Mindful Energy Links

The concept of a beautiful vinyasa in yoga asana practice, creates the vision of a yoga practitioner moving seamlessly between yoga postures with awareness and fluid grace. This is definitely part of the definition of fluid vinyasa in yoga and yet the concept can reach far beyond, to include mindful awareness in all aspects of your life. This heightened perception of higher consciousness expands outward to inspire enhanced awareness and productivity of your daily thoughts and actions. Studying the benefits and categories of vinyasa and how to use them can assist you greatly in your own yoga practice and becomes a valuable tool for teachers too.

Definition of Vinyasa

Vinyasa (*vi-nyaah-sa*) derived from a Sanskrit term and is often embraced in relation to certain styles, or techniques of modern day yoga. If we look much deeper into the term vinyasa, the word may be broken down into its Sanskrit roots which will greatly assist in realizing its true meaning. *Nyasa* translates as meaning "to place," or, "to step" and *vi* translates as meaning "in a special" or "specific way." The Sanskrit words often have several different meanings as the word *vinyasa* also depicts slightly different meanings.

Vinyasa: In the book, "Heart of Yoga," T.K.V. Desikachar, a very popular and highly respected guru defines vinyasa yoga as: *Karma* = Step, *vi* = in a special way, *nyasa* = to place. This implies the conscious energy connection between your body, mind, breath, and life force, which then creates your karma and ultimately becomes your path in life.

WHAT IS / YOGA VINYASA IN PRACTICE?

Yoga vinyasa in practice; is a conscious energy connection between yoga asanas and can also be a link between moments, or concepts in time. Yoga means union, yoking, or to bring together in harmony. In the yoga community, vinyasa yoga usually describes a system, or style of yoga asana practice, although "yoga vinyasa" in itself is not a system yet a way of practicing. There are two different concepts to practicing vinyasa: 1) the visual or physical vinyasa concept, and 2) the mental, unseen, or energetic vinyasa concept. Embracing both concepts is the appropriate meaning of conscious and holistic yoga practice.

1) **The Physical Vinyasa Concept:** This represents various formal manors to transition between yoga asana. In the vinyasa yoga systems you will be given a specific body movement, to be used in conjunction with synchronized breath and mental awareness. This application of vinyasa becomes much like an electrical wire connecting power between cities.

2) **The Energetic or Invisible Vinyasa Concept**: You will become one with energy, through the avenue of mental awareness and breathe to create a fluid energetic practice. Of course, as I mentioned previously, you can and should learn to use aspects from both concepts of vinyasa yoga and in the end will find the physical and energetic aspects will complement one another.

Benefits of Vinyasa — In Yoga and Life
   1. Creates Internal Heat
   2. Distributes Prana (Energy)
   3. Clears your Energy Field
   4. Inspires Moving Meditation
   5. Balances Body and Mind

The vinyasa connects postures, thoughts or energy together, creating internal heat which helps distribute pranic energy throughout your body as it clears your energy field for a new asana. In addition, the fluid manor in which you move your body with focused breathing also affects the mind in a positive way creating greater awareness and perception, inspiring balance.

Think beyond the generic phrase "vinyasa yoga" as just a link between asana and reflect upon larger aspects, far beyond the physical yoga asana practice. Symbolically, the vinyasa of your life is a river flowing to the sea, a conscious connection between moments and events in time. Once you see the larger picture, the awareness you create in your yoga asana practice can expand to touch every aspect of your daily life.

When you find a way to embrace greater awareness in your daily life then you are more productive and make better decisions. The new found awareness can be very advantageous in making better choices in nutrition, relationships and lifestyle. This same mindset over time creates higher consciousness, enhanced spirituality, and inner peace.

Throwing a Pebble in the Pond

Your whole life is similar to throwing a pebble into a quiet pond, which creates ripples; these ripples are gradually expanding to touch the distant shores, even after the pebble has gone. In your life, what you say and what you do, how you act and what you represent creates ripples in time, touching Humans in future generations long after you are gone. Conscious yoga practice inspires conscious daily action, which in turn touches all life in a positive way.

CATEGORIZING VINYASA (HARD AND SOFT)

Hard and Soft Vinyasa:
1. Hard Vinyasa - (More muscle resistance / More challenging)
2. Soft Vinaysa - (Less muscle resistance / Less challenging)

In Pioneering Vinyasa Yoga, there are two basic types of vinyasa. Each vinyasa has its own character and is appropriate for different phases of your practice. Some vinyasas need to be very strenuous in order generate body heat. These vinyasa demand more muscular work and are designed to be more active. I call these hard, or "hot vinyasa." Other vinyasas are designed to be less demanding on your muscles and create less heat, yet they still build energy and power.

These less strenuous vinyasa I call soft, or "cool vinyasa" which are much less challenging movements between your yoga postures.

Every level of practice should strive to include a balance of both hard and soft vinyasa. A wise yogi or yogini might plan on using the softer vinyasa with one practice and the harder vinyasa with the next practice. The sage advice, at any level of practice is to incorporate both (challenging / hard) and (non-challenging / soft) vinyasa with your regular yoga practice and occasionally practice your yoga without vinyasa.

The title *Hatha Yoga* relates to anyone "practicing yoga asana," in any style and level of intensity. Breaking down the word *hatha*, the preface *ha*, means "masculine," or "sun." The preface *tha* means "feminine," or "moon"; the word *yoga* means "union, bringing together," or "yoking." Hatha Yoga is the union of hard and soft concepts, inspiring a holistic balance.

HOW TO USE VINYASA

Learning the Sadhana Vinyasa / Connecting Links

Vinyasas are the heart and soul of the Sadhana Vinyasa Yoga program. You use the vinyasa as a means of entering and exiting each yoga posture and as a path to mindful practice. These connecting movements prevent any break in the energy flow of your routine and create a smooth graceful flow. For example, if you are in a seated posture and you need to go into a standing pose, you can scramble to your feet, frantically tug at your workout clothes, and slowly with the grace of a drunken elephant, put yourself into position. This cute example is a poor representation of yoga vinyasa and asana practice.

On the other hand, if you move mindfully with smooth connections in your vinyasa, you increase your body heat and awareness of energy, as you maintain the power of your routine's momentum. By doing your vinyasa correctly, you will take on the beauty and power of nature. Practicing yoga **without** awareness will result in your routine being scattered, disconnected, and much less effective.

Important Note - In the beginning, you may choose to practice my yoga routines without the use of vinyasa, however in time as you become familiar with the asana; I suggest you embrace the suggested vinyasa for each separate asana. The use of my unique vinyasa system will greatly reward you with enhanced physical, mental and spiritual awareness and create the amazingly harmonious flow of this beautiful practice.

Moving with Energy

In Sadhana Vinyasa Yoga, you will learn to go with the natural lines of energy, rather than fighting against them. Natural lines of energy refer to the flow of energy which creates the least resistance or stress within your posture or flowing link, as related to the individual needs. The natural lines of energy can be affected by internal and external forces; I refer to this as surrendering to the posture. You will learn to avoid fighting against your yoga practice, yet to go with energy and make friends with your yoga pose. For example, if you are doing a Downward Facing Dog Posture you can fight against the pull of gravity, or relax and allow the gravity to gently lengthen your neck and upper back, at the same time becoming neutral and allowing the earth's energy to run through your body. In this manor, you learn to use the power of the whole universe to work with you rather than against you.

Speed or Pace of Vinyasa

How fast you move through your vinyasa also affects the cardio and muscle resistance and qualities of your practice. Surprisingly, the slower you move in your vinyasa practice, the greater the quality of muscle resistance will be with less cardio. Moving at a slower rate in your vinyasa, you remain in the muscle resistance zone longer than when you're moving very quickly. On the other hand, when you move faster you create more cardio while using less muscle resistance.

For example, if two students practiced a Sun Salutation, the student who moved slower and finished last would achieve a greater muscular workout. The one who moved quicker would be increasing the heart rate, so a balanced practice should embrace both concepts.

One of the key factors in determining just how much of an anaerobic workout you will get is the vinyasa, or linking movements between your yoga postures. You can choose a vinyasa that is very physically demanding (hot vinyasa), or you can choose a vinyasa that is very low energy (soft vinyasa). The difference between these choices is dramatic, and again, the choice is up to you. You can choose the harder vinyasas, the softer vinyasas, or use a bit of both.

Being Here Now / Awareness and Spirituality

The purely physical aspect of vinyasa is simply a work-out, yet the underlying energy which allows you to move is called prana, or life force energy. This invisible energy is present in all living things. The greater concept of a yoga vinyasa is to be aware of the energy behind the vinyasa, which inspires a greater awareness in all of life. Blindly racing through your vinyasa for a great work out and try to hurry on toward the next asana, so you can get there first, lacks awareness and does not represent the true meaning of yoga vinyasa, it is just fitness. The same concept can be used in any other physical and mental activities.

If you can, be "here and now" to embrace an acute awareness of energy in your vinyasa, this can then inspire a more spiritual practice, which can mean different things to different people. You may feel spirituality is a natural bond with nature or faith in a greater power, or perhaps a union of universal energy within your own body and mind. This is a personal matter and the answers will surely come when the student is ready.

Simply described, you can manifest a more genuine flow in vinyasa, if your mind travels with you. Remember these masterful words in life: "the journey is everything." In your yoga practice, ***don't just go through the motions***, strive to be present and in doing so embrace a sense of sacred spirituality (Positive thoughts, kindness, non-violence and gratitude).

Once you commit yourself to this concept of yoga practice, many answers will come to you. In time you will discover that your yoga practice also affects your whole life in a positive way. Your daily life will take on an essence of controlled energy flow. Yoga is an internal practice with external results touching every aspect of your whole life in a positive way. In yoga, this is called harmony within!

Moving Meditation – The Ultimate Vinyasa Flow

Your practice of yoga is for you and ultimately it should be something you feel very comfortable with. As in all things, you've got to start somewhere! Do you remember the first time you rode a bicycle, drove a car, or went surfing? It seemed like an enormous task to master any of these activities: I'm sure you felt that you would never find them relaxing or comfortable? Luckily, once you understand the basics, all these activities just became second nature.

You will find the same to be true of your Sadhana Vinyasa Yoga practice, in time all the details will become second nature and you can just move with the natural flow of energy, like a surfer riding the energy of a beautiful wave. I remember when I was a struggling beginner in my yoga practice and I tried fixating too hard on all the minor details. I really had a miserable time at my yoga, and it was more like work than something relaxing and enjoyable.

Then, one day I decided to just let go of all the details and practice some easy and fun yoga outdoors. It was a really wonderful experience… being able to free my spirit and practice yoga. Gradually I embraced all the concepts and details of a good yoga practice. Today, my yoga practice is of genuine quality, yet very free flowing and comfortable, embracing the essential balance of strength and softness. Physically I am amazingly strong, mentally I have a perceptive mind, and spiritually I am at peace with myself and with my place in the universe.

Becoming one … Yoga as Energy

The ultimate in Sadhana Vinyasa Yoga asana practice is to embrace all your connecting movements as a moving meditation. As you gain confidence, strength, and greater awareness with your practice, you will strive toward having a deep sense of awareness in all aspects of your movements, yet with effortless fluidity.

Details for Vinyasa: (Connecting Energy Links)

Details and instructions will be given for each vinyasa along with suggested use and cautions. The photos will also demonstrate visual flow of the vinyasa.

Choices of Vinyasa

In this chapter I list the most practical vinyasas which can be used with a variety of yoga asanas and styles of practice. You should try to eventually use my suggested vinyasa for each pose, yet sometimes choose to practice yoga asana without vinyasa taking a rest and time to reflect.

(Ex = Exhale / In = Inhale)

THE VINYASA OF LIFE

Mindful awareness; a rivers journey

To the sea

Vin # 1 – Wheel Vinyasa *(Chakrasana)*   *Moderate – Some Power*

Chakra means "wheel" and *Asana* means "pose". In this vinyasa you will roll backward resembling a wheel. Inspired from Ashtanga Yoga and also used in tumbling and gymnastics classes.

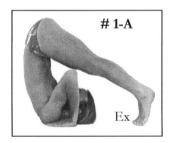

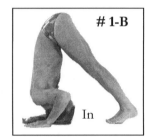

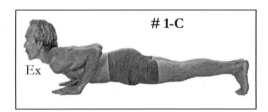

Use of Vinyasa: Most often used only as an exit of poses when lying on your back. Such as: Shoulder Stand. **Modify (#1-A / #1-B) – elevate shoulders on a folded blanket).**

Cautions: (Injury of: Neck, Wrist, and Shoulders – plus Pregnancy).

Instructions: Vin # 1 - Wheel Vinyasa (Pg 52)

1. From a position lying on your back, exhale bend your knees in toward your chest, as you roll backward, with hands under shoulders **(photo # 1-A).**

2. Once your hands touch the floor push downward away from shoulders, as you reach for the floor with your feet **(photo # 1-B).** Ideally you will take a soft landing in Four Limbed Staff Pose **(photo # 1-C).** Then take Up-dog to Down-dog.

Vin # 2-A – Vinyasa Jump Back (Part 1)   *Difficult – More Power*

The inspiration of this vinyasa in yoga was from Ashtanga – the technique and concept is also used in power yoga, fitness and gymnastics. **(Modify 2-A, B - Place hands on blocks).**

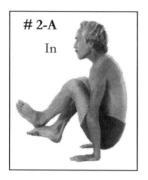

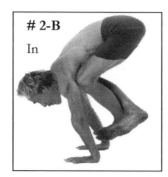

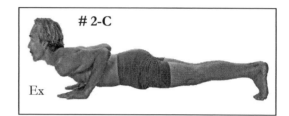

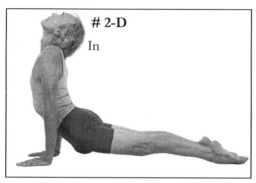

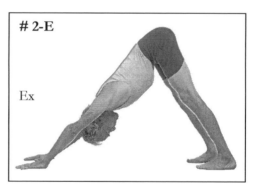

Vin # 2-B – Vinyasa Jump Forward (Part 2)   *Difficult – More Power*

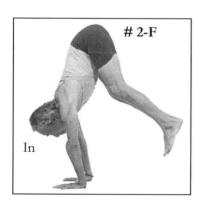

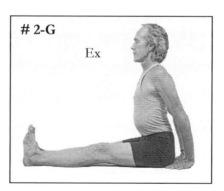

Vin # 2-C – Vinyasa Jump to Stand (Part 3)   *Difficult – More Power*

The inspiration of this vinyasa in yoga was from Ashtanga – the concept and technique is also used in power yoga, fitness and gymnastics programs. If you want to take a more powerful link to standing, or for arm balancing practice this is a good choice.

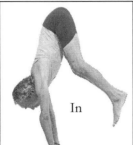
2-H

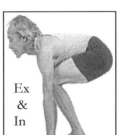
2-I

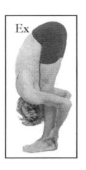
2-J

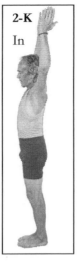
2-K

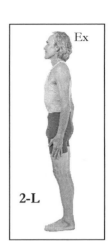
2-L

Use of Vinyasa:

(Part 1) - Can be used when you want to move out of a seated pose and add extra challenge, more strength and build more heat with a vinyasa. **Modify - place hands on blocks.**

(Part 2) - Can be used, when you want to move into a seated pose and add extra challenge, more strength and build more heat with a vinyasa. **Modify - place hands on blocks.**

(Part 3) - Can be used, to move into a standing pose, or arm balanced and add extra challenge, more strength and build more heat with a vinyasa. **Modify - just step forward instead of jump.**

Cautions: Injury of: Wrists, Elbows and Shoulders – plus Pregnancy Precautions.

Instructions: Vin # 2 – (Part 1 – 3) Jump Back / Forward / Standing – (Pg 53- 54)

1. Start from a cross-legged seated position; now place your hands on the floor to the side of your hips. Now inhale as you pull your knees up toward your chest, pushing down with hands and lifting with abdominal muscles, as you engage your bandhas **(photo # 2-A).**

2. Now lean forward, lift with your hips and drop head downward, as you lift backward and upward **(photo # 2-B).** To modify - allow toes to touch the floor and push.

3. On your exhale, release bandhas and land softly into Four Limbed Staff Pose **(photo # 2-C).**

4. Now inhale and move to Upward Facing Dog Pose **(photo # 2-D)** and then exhale to Downward Facing Dog, **(photo # 2-E).**

5. **Vin # 2-B, 2-C – (Part 2 and 3)** Depending on where you are going – you can jump back through to a seated position **(photo # 2-F and 2-G),** or jump to standing position **(photo # 2-H to 2-L),** or you can just (Relax in Down Dog, or Childs Pose).

Vin # 3 – Flying Vinyasa   *Difficult – More Power*

Popular in Ashtanga and Power yoga - this vinyasa inspired by the Flying Insect Pose and when you master this vinyasa you will feel as if you can fly back on your wings.

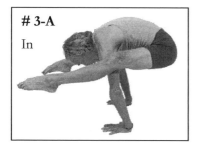
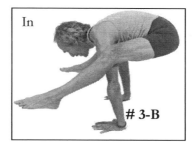
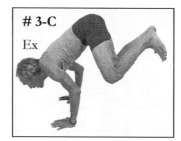

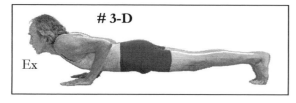

Modify – Place blocks under your hands, or just step back / no jump.

Use of Vinyasa:

Can be used with most any asana when you start in a seated position, or many of the arm balances poses will do well as an exit, or entrance vinyasa.

Cautions: (Injury of: Wrist, Elbows and Shoulders – plus Pregnancy).

Instructions: <u>Flying Vin - # 3 (Pg 55)</u>

1. From Flying Insect Pose, push down with your hands, stay strong in the core, as in **(Photo # 3-A),** when you inhale lift your hips and lower feet **(photo # 3-B).**

2. Once you have the altitude, lift legs off your arms, bending knees slightly as you drop your head and push your feet backward **(photo # 3-C)** and land softly into Four Limbed Staff Pose **(photo # 3-D). Advanced** can go to handstand then to Four Limbed Staff.

Vin # 4 – Missing Link Vinyasa (Part 1 - Up)   *Soft – Less Power*

After years of practicing yoga, I always thought there was something missing! Yoga needed a soft vinyasa to standing and back down again. Therefore, with much practice and study of energy lines - I created **The Missing Link** vinyasa. This is very soft, gentle and can be modified with props to suit your needs. **(Missing Link Vinyasa / Begin on next page).**

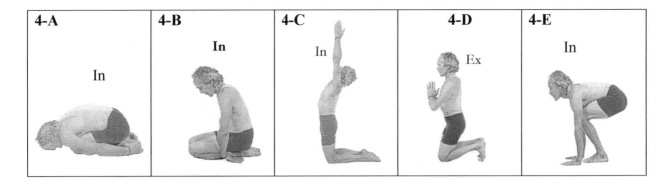

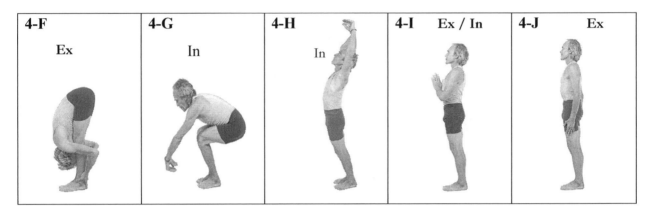

Use of Vinyasa:

Can be used as a soft, gentle and meditative link to connect seated poses to standing and used in **(Vin # 5)** you can go back to seated from standing.

Modify and Prop Use – Place a folded blanket under your knees and **(In steps 4-D and 4-E),** place your hands onto blocks to assist with standing up. Instead of starting on knees – **Start with (Step 4-E)** – yet sitting on two blocks with knees bent – then follow same instructions to finish.

Cautions: (Injury of: Knees and Ankles).

Instructions: <u>Missing Link - Vin # 4 (Part 1 Up) – (Pg 55 - 57)</u>

1. Start in Folded Leaf Pose **(photo 4-A),** then inhale and begin to lift your torso up off your thighs. Stay relaxed and uncoil one vertebra at a time **(photo 4-B).**
2. Now lift your head upward and expand your chest, as you lift your hips off your heels, placing palms together up over your head as you gaze upward **(photo # 4-C).**
3. Start your exhalation as you flex your feet and lower hands in prayer fashion over your heart **(photo # 4-D).**

4. Now place your hands on the floor, with knees bent, as you move weight onto your feet **(photo # 4-E)**. Remain in Photo 4-E and take a slow deep inhalation, then as you exhale move into a standing forward bend and exhale **(photo # 4-F)**.

5. Bend your knees as you as you start to inhale, flowing your arms forward with soft wrist **(photo # 4-G)**. Continue the same fluid motion as you come to a standing position, arching backward slightly, with arms up over your head **(photo # 4-H)**.

6. Begin your exhalation, as you lower your hands in prayer fashion down over your heart **(photo # 4-I)**. Take a slow deep inhalation, then as you exhale lower hands by your sides into Mountain Pose and relax **(photo # 4-J)**.

Vin # 5 – Missing Link Vinyasa – (Part 2 - Down)   *Soft – Less Power*

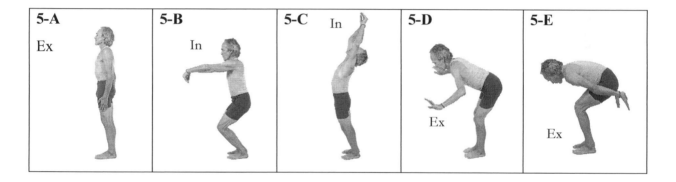

➢ You have the option to finish in seated or kneeling posture, **(photo # 5-H, 5-I, 5-J)**.

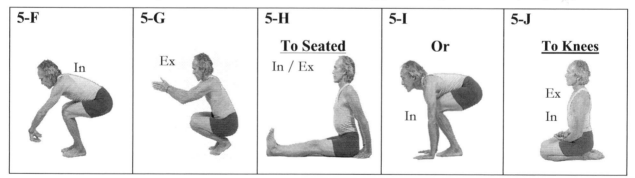

Use of Vinyasa:

Can be used as a soft, gentle and meditative link to connect standing poses to seated poses and in (Vin # 4) you can go back to standing from seated.

Modify and Prop Use – **(In steps 5-G, 5-H, 5-I)** place your hands onto blocks to assist with seated or kneeling position. In **(photo 5-J) t**he Kneeling Position – sit on a block between your ankles.

Cautions: Injury of: Knees and Ankles.

Instructions: <u>Missing Link - Vin # 4 (Part 2 Down) – (Pg 57, 58)</u>

1. Start in Mountain Pose **(photo 5-A)** with an exhale, then as you inhale begin to lift your arms in a flowing motion, as you bend your knees slightly **(photo # 5-B)**.
2. Continue your inhalation, lifting arms up over your head, as you arch gently backward **(photo # 5-C)**. Now begin your exhalation as you bend forward at the waist and circle arms outward and downward **(photo # 5-D)**.
3. Continue the exhalation; try to straighten your legs, dropping you head and shoulders downward toward your feet, as you lift your hips upward. Lift arms straight behind your back **(photo # 5-E)**.
4. Start the inhalation, as you bend your knees and flow your arms forward, with wrist soft. Begin to lift your head and find you balance **(photo # 5-F)**.
5. Allow your heels to come up slightly, as you place hands together in prayer and get ready to move to a seated position as you exhale **(photo # 5-G)**.
6. Finish in a seated position **(photo 5-H)** take one complete breath and relax. If you prefer to finish on a position resting on your knees **(Skip steps 5-G and 5-H)** and instead follow steps **(5-I and 5-J)**.

Vin # 6 – Easy Breezy Vinyasa   *Soft – Less Power*

I came up with this vinyasa, as a very gentle and easy way to link seated poses without expending a lot of energy. In these movements you will conserve energy and still create a continuous flow and gentle counter stretch.

Use of Vinyasa:
This gentle vinyasa works with any ground based, non-standing poses. For example, if you have several seated poses in a routine, you can use this vinyasa between poses or right and left sides of poses to create a nice gentle flow.

Cautions: Hip injury or Lower Back issues.

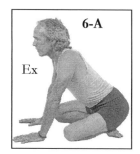

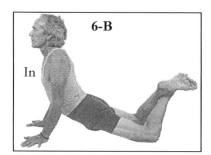

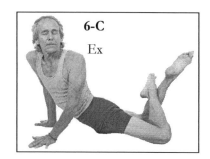

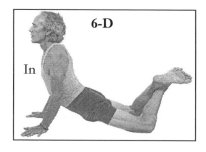

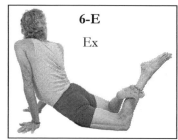

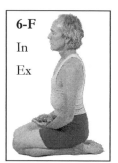

Instructions: Easy Breezy - Vin # 6 (Pg 58, 59)

1. Start in a seated cross-legged position with hands resting on the ground in front of your knees **(photo # 6-A)** exhale and relax.

2. Inhale, keeping knees spread wide and ankles crossed, as you slowly walk hands forward and allow hips to stretch toward the floor **(photo # 6-B)**.

3. Now exhale and twist your torso to the left **(photo # 6-C)**. Then inhale and return to the middle position **(photo # 6-D)**.

4. Then repeat by twisting your torso to the right, **(photo # 6-E)** as you exhale. Then return to the middle position for one more inhale **(photo # 6-B)**.

5. To finish - exhale as you move back to a kneeling position **(photo # 6-F)**, or Childs Pose or back to the seated position you started from.

6. **Option – Inhale to Cobra Pose (Pg 167) and exhale to Childs Pose (Pg 94)** this is also a very nice vinyasa option and easy to practice.

Vin # 7 – Eagle Wings Vinyasa *Soft – Less Power*

After many years of practicing yoga in nature, I gained a close bond with animals and birds, I could actually hear the message in the wind and feel the heart-beat of earth itself. In this asana you will resemble an eagle stretching its wings before flight.

Practical Benefits:

In this vinyasa you release tension from your wrist, elbows and shoulders, as well as creating a very meditative, sacred and honored atmosphere as you enter your asana.

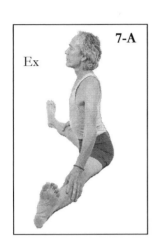

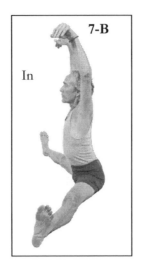

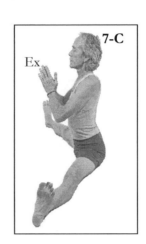

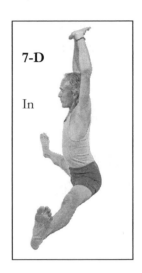

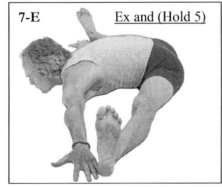

Use of Vinyasa:

This gentle and sacred vinyasa works very well with the leg stretch progression, inhale lift your wings, then exhale honor yourself and pay gratitude. Then inhale again to release tension from wrist and exhale as you enter your asana.

(This is a demo pose – yet this Vinyasa may be used to enter many poses)

Cautions: Hip injury or Lower Back issues.

Instructions: Eagle Wings - Vin # 7 (Pg 59 - 61)

1. Start in a Seated Angle **(Pg 87, # 2-A)** then split legs wide, hands resting on your legs as you embrace good posture **(photo # 7-A)**. Less flexible bend knees with blocks under knees and sit on folded blanket. Relax for 1- 2 complete breaths.

2. Then on an inhalation lift your arms out to the sides of your torso and up over your head, with soft wrist – as if moving under water **(photo # 7-B)**.

3. Now exhale and lower your hands in prayer fashion down in front of your heart **(photo # 7-C)**.

4. Next you will interlace your fingers and start to rotate your hands with palms facing outward and upward, as you inhale and stretch hands and arms up over your head **(photo # 6-D).**

5. The last step you will exhale and move slowly into your asana and hold for 5- breaths **(photo # 7-E).** – (Keep in mind, this is only a demo pose – you can use this technique with many other seated poses, kneeling poses and some standing poses.

Vin # 8 – Sun Dial Vinayasa   *Soft – Less Power*

If you look at the final pose, it resembles a sun dial, hence the name was born. This fluid vinyasa is similar to the energy you create with a moving meditation, as in Thi Chi, in addition to opening hips and relaxing arms for your next asana.

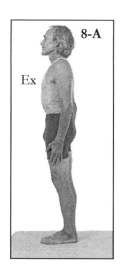

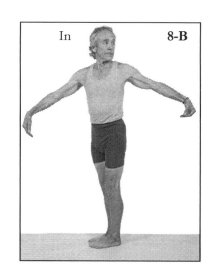

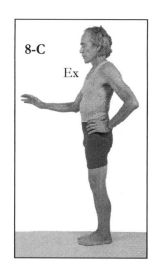

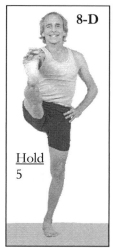

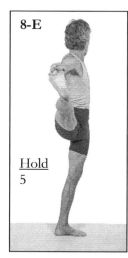

Use of Vinyasa:
This very fluid and meditative vinyasa works with Sun Dial pose and various other standing poses and will help with coordination and balance.

Cautions:
Ankle Injury, or balance issues.

Modify: Use wall for support and strap to extend reach for toes.

Instructions: <u>Sun Dial - Vin # 8 (Pg 61, 62)</u>

1. Start in Mountain Pose **(photo # 8-A)**, take one slow deep breath and relax. On your next inhalation slowly move your right arm forward and your left arm backward in a fluid relaxed motion, with your gaze slightly behind you and hips open to the left **(photo # 8-B)**.

2. Continue your inhalation as you lift your arms higher, keeping wrists soft and relaxed.

3. Begin your exhalation as you lower your arms and square your hips to the front, allowing your left hand to rest on your left hip and your right arm bent at the elbow, as you prepare to grasp your right toes **(photo # 8-C)**, or **(Less flexible just hold your right knee)**.

4. Bend your right knee and grasp your big toe, with the thumb and first two fingers of your right hand, as you extend the right leg forward **(photo # 8-D)**. *Remember this is just a demo pose, you can use this vinyasa for other standing poses as well.*

5. You may also continue and move the leg to the right side **(photo # 8-E)**.

Vin # 9 – Chi Flow Vinayasa *Soft – Less Power*

This vinyasa is similar to the manor that students of Tai Chi learn how to feel energy and move with the flow of life force.

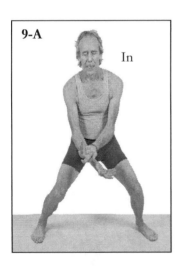
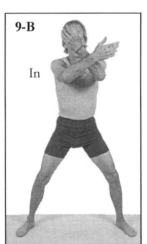
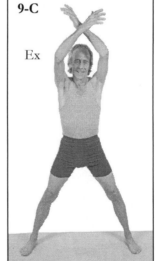
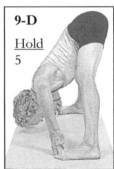

Use of Vinyasa:

This soft and yet powerful vinyasa works well with the Expanded Foot Pose sequence and many other standing poses, as a way to move energy with your asana and create a meditative atmosphere. This vinyasa works well to enter and also exit many standing asana.

Cautions: Knee and Ankle injury, or Lower Back pain.

Instructions: <u>**Chi Flow - Vin # 9 (Pg 62, 63)**</u>

1. Start in a standing position with feet parallel and (1 – 4 feet apart) depending on which asana you are using this with. Then start your inhalation as you bend your knees and cross your arms in front of your thighs, pelvis and lower abdominals, try to feel as if you are moving through liquid **(photo # 9-A).**

2. Continue your inhalation as you lift your arms up in in front of your chest and shoulders, drawing the energy to the upper body **(photo # 9-B).**

3. Now lift arms up over your head, begin your exhalation releasing the energy **(photo # 9-C).** Then bend forward at the waist and slowly move into the asana of your choice **(photo # 9-D).**

<u>**Vin # 10 – Side Angle Vinyasa (Part 1)**</u> *Soft – Less Power*

In this vinyasa you will learn to move with prana and become one with the life force, as you also embrace a very meditative atmosphere.

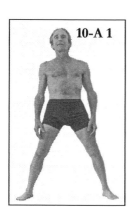
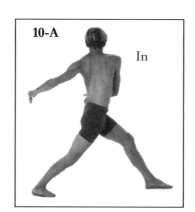
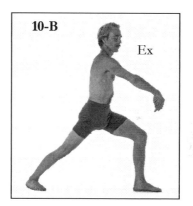

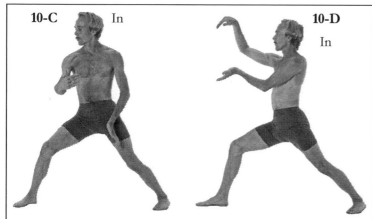
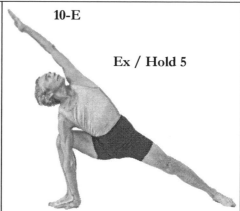

Cautions: Knee, or Ankle injury and Lower Back pain.

Use of Vinyasa:

This soft and yet powerful vinyasa works well with the sequence of Side Angle Pose and Twisted Side Angle Pose. The fluid lines create a beautiful progression, with a meditative atmosphere, as you move like a river flowing to the sea. This flow gently opens shoulders, spine, wrists and ankles, as you enhance balance and coordination.

Instructions: Side Angle Vin # 10 (Part 1 - Pg 63 - 64)

1. Start in a very wide standing position with feet parallel (3 – 4 feet apart) and arms resting by your sides **(photo # 10-A 1)**. Then inhale as you pivot your torso and feet to the left, at the same time, moving arms in a sweeping motion to the left, with your weight distributed evenly between both feet and your gaze in the direction of the twist **(photo # 10-A).**

2. Now start your exhalation, as you softly sweep your arms to the right side, pivoting on your feet and lunging deeply into the left knee, as you bring your weight forward **(photo # 10-B) .**

3. On your next inhalation, slowly begin to twist your whole torso to the right, leading with your right arm and gently pushing with your left hand, as you begin to shift the weight from your left leg to your right leg **(photo # 10-C).**

4. Then continue your inhalation, as you lift your left hand to heart level, with palm facing upward and lift your right hand to your third eye, with palm facing downward **(photo # 10-D).** Now begin to shift your weight more to your right leg.

5. Begin your exhalation - slowly moving toward the asana, as you lower your right arm down to the floor and your left arm up extending up over head, on the same line of your torso, as you enter your asana **(photo # 10-E).** Less flexible... simply rest your right elbow on your right thigh, or use a yoga block under your right hand.

Vin # 11 – Twisted Side Angle Vinyasa (Part 2)   *Soft – Less Power*

This vinyasa is the sibling of (Side Angle Vinyasa) only this time you add a nice twist to the final asana. In this vinyasa you will learn to move with prana and become one with the life force, as you also embrace a very meditative atmosphere.

Use of Vinyasa:

This soft and yet powerful vinyasa works well with the sequence of Side Angle Pose and Twisted Side Angle Pose. The fluid lines create a beautiful progression, with a meditative atmosphere, as you move like a river flowing to the sea. This flow gently opens shoulders, spine, wrist and ankles, as you enhance balance and coordination.

Cautions: Knee, or ankle injury and lower back pain.

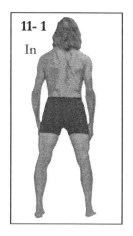

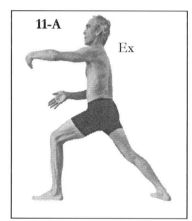

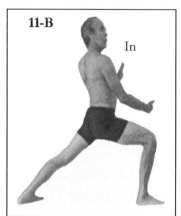

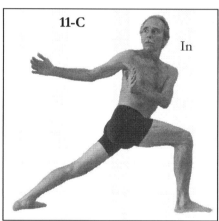

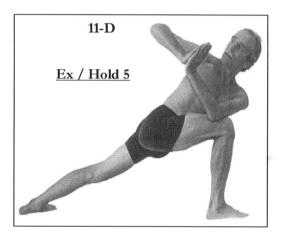

Instructions: Twisted Side Angle - Vin # 11 (Part 2 - Pg 64 - 66)

1. Start in a very wide standing position with feet parallel (3 – 4 feet apart) and arms resting by your sides **(photo # 11-1)**. Begin your exhalation pivoting your torso and feet to the left, at the same time - moving arms in a sweeping motion to the left, as you bend into your left knee with your weight mostly on your left foot. Your gaze is out parallel to the ground and thoughts relaxed **(photo # 11-A)**.

2. Now begin your inhalation, slowly sweeping your arms to the right side, leading with your right arm and pushing with your left hand, as you move your weight from your left foot to your right foot **(photo # 11-B)**. Keep your torso upright and shoulders back and gaze parallel to the ground.

3. Continue your inhalation as you lower your left shoulder toward your right thigh, at the same time moving your right arm backward and upward, with hands about 3-feet apart

and palms facing one another **(photo # 11-C).** Lunge to a 90-Degree angle on your right knee, with abdominals engaged.

4. Now begin your exhalation as you lower your left elbow down, to rest on your right knee, bringing palms together in prayer fashion over your heart. Strive to draw one line of energy from your extended left foot through your torso and out the top of your head **(photo # 11-D).**

Vin # 12 – Short Jump Vinyasa   *Soft to Moderate – Less Power*

This vinyasa is used with a fluid manor to jump or step your feet a short distance apart. The technique is used often in Ashtanga Yoga and Power Yoga.

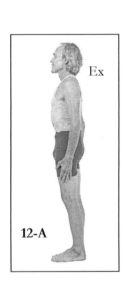
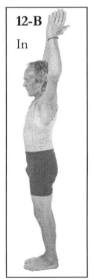
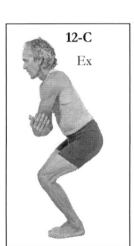
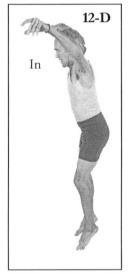
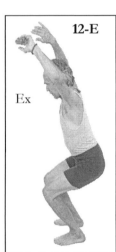

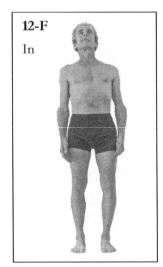

Use of Vinyasa:

This vinyasa helps to generate heat and to create a fluid connection in many standing asanas. Several styles use this vinyasa to get in and out of *padangusthasasna* and *pada hastasana*.

Cautions: Knee, or Ankle injury, Lower Back pain and Pregnancy.

Modify: Step instead of jumping for a slower pace and lower impact.

Instructions: Short Jump - Vin # 12 (Pg 66 - 67)

1. Start from a standing positon in Mountain Pose **(photo 12-A)** with feet together and hands by your sides, then take one complete inhalation and exhalation.

2. On your next inhalation, lift your arms up over your head with palms together **(photo # 12-B).**

3. Then exhale, bending your knees and crossing your arms in front of your abdominals, as you prepare to jump **(photo # 12-C).**

4. Now inhale, as you thrust your arms up over your head and jump upward **(photo # 12-D).**

5. Begin your exhalation, landing softly, with feet about 1 foot apart, as you bend the knees, lower your hips and lift arms up over your shoulders **(photo # 12-E).**

6. Continue the exhalation, as you return to standing in Mountain Pose, only this time with feet about one foot apart **(photo # 12-F).**

7. **Lesser, or softer Option** – Step your feet apart, instead of jumping.

Vin # 13 – Wide Jump Vinyasa   *Soft to Moderate – Some Power*

This vinyasa is the sibling of the Short Jump Vinyasa, only this time you are taking a half turn to the side and landing with feet in a much wider position. In this vinyasa you will learn to create a flowing link in order to stand sideways on your mat.

Use of Vinyasa:

This (soft to moderate) vinyasa works well with the sequence of moving from a standing pose with a narrow stance and then transitioning to a standing pose with a wider stance.

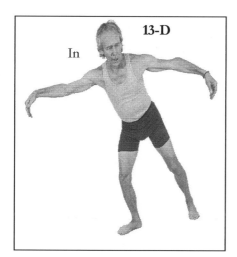
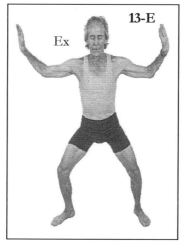
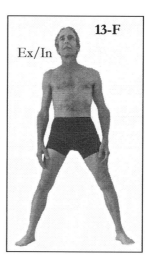

Cautions: Knee, or Ankle injury, Lower Back pain and Pregnancy.

Instructions: **Wide Jump - Vin # 13 (Pg 67 - 68)**

1. Start from a standing positon in Mountain Pose **(Pg 66, photo 12-A)** with feet together and hands by your sides, then take one complete inhalation and exhalation.

2. On your next inhalation, lift your arms up over your head with palms together **(Pg 66, photo # 12-B).**

3. Then exhale, bending your knees and crossing your arms in front of your abdominals, as you prepare to step or jump to your left side **(Pg 66, photo # 12-C).**

4. Now inhale, as you thrust your arms up over your head and then step, pivot or jump to your left side, with a very wide stance **(Pg 67, photo # 13-D).**

5. Begin your exhalation, landing softly, with feet about 3-4 feet apart, as you bend the knees, lower your hips and lift your arms softly, out to the sides of your shoulders. With palms facing outward **(Pg 67, photo # 13-E).**

6. Continue your exhalation as you slowly stand up and relax, only now you are in a wide stance and facing sideways you your mat **(Pg 67, photo # 13-F).**

7. **Important Note** – The next time you use this vinyasa – jump, step, or pivot to the right side to create balance.

Vin # 14 – Triangle Vinyasa   *Soft – Less Power*

After years of yoga practice, I created this vinyasa, which is much more than just a link between poses. The Triangle Vinyasa will lengthen the spine; open your hips and shoulders, as it creates smooth meditative lines of energy into and out of Triangle Pose.

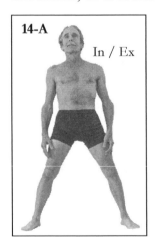
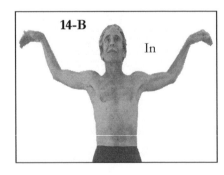
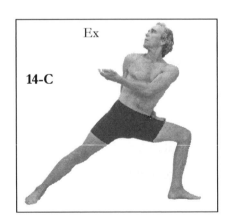

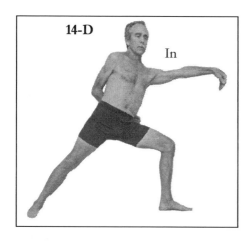

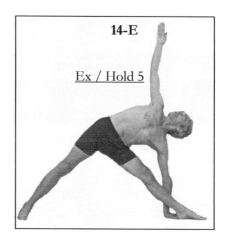

Use of Vinyasa:

This soft and yet powerful vinyasa works as an excellent, high quality vinyasa to enter and exit Triangle pose and can be used with Half Moon Pose and several other standing asanas.

Cautions: Knee, or Ankle injury, Lower Back pain, Eye injury.

Instructions: **Triangle Vin # 14 (Pg 68 - 69)**

1. Start with a wide stance in a standing position **(Pg 68, photo # 14-A)** then take one complete breath, inhale and exhale.

2. On your next inhalation, softy lift your arms out to the sides of your torso and up over your head, with wrist bend and palms facing downward **(Pg 68, photo # 14-B).**

3. Begin your exhalation as you pivot your left foot to the left and lunge deeply into the left knee. At the same time sweep your left arm in front of your torso, as you move your right arm back behind your lower back, opening your hips, with your gaze over your right shoulder looking backward **(Pg 68, photo # 14-C).**

4. Now inhale reaching forward with your left arm, as you begin to straighten your left leg **(Pg 69, photo # 14-D).**

5. Then begin your exhalation as you move slowly into your Triangle Pose and relax for 5 breaths **(photo # 14-E**

6. **(Pg 69, photo # 14-E).** When finished, exhale bending your left knee, then inhale and return to standing, then practice the same technique on the opposite side.

7. **Triangle Option** – Rest left hand on your lower leg, or use a block under your left hand, or practice with a wall behind your back.

Vin # 15 – Revolved Triangle Vinyasa   *Soft – Less Power*

This vinyasa is much more than just a link between poses. The Revolved Triangle Vinyasa will expand the chest; open the shoulders inspire the hips to relax, in addition to embracing a fluid and meditative connection into and out of this asana.

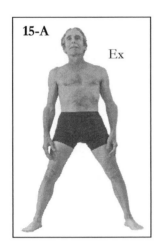

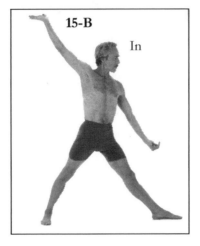

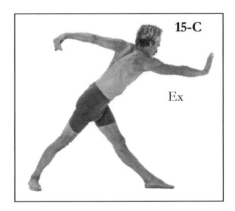

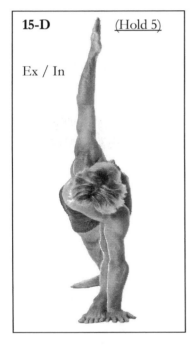

Use of Vinyasa:

This soft and yet powerful vinyasa works as an excellent, high quality vinyasa to enter and exit the Revolved Triangle Pose and can be used with a variety of other standing asanas.

Cautions:

Knee, Ankle, Hip, or Eye injury.

Modify Final Pose:

Use a block under your supporting right hand, or rest your right forearm on your left thigh.

Instructions: Revolved Triangle - Vin # 15 (Pg 70 - 71)

1. Start with a wide stance in a standing position **(Pg 70, photo # 15-A)** and take one slow deep exhalation and relax.

2. On your next inhalation begin to pivot your left foot to the left side as you lower your left arm and lift your right arm, in a windmill fashion **(Pg 70, photo # 15-B).**

3. Start your exhalation, as you continue the circular motion of your arms, lowering your right arm and lifting your left arm, with wrist soft. Begin to square your hips to the left as you lean your torso to the left **(Pg 70, photo # 15-C).**

4. Continue your exhalation as you move into the Revolved Triangle Pose **(Pg 70, photo # 15-D)** with your right hand resting on the outside of your left foot and hips squared, dropping your right shoulder down and lifting your left shoulder upward, with your gaze up toward your left hand.

5. **Modification** - Rest your right hand on a yoga block, either in front or behind your left foot. You may also bend your left knee slightly and allow the hips to be less squared.

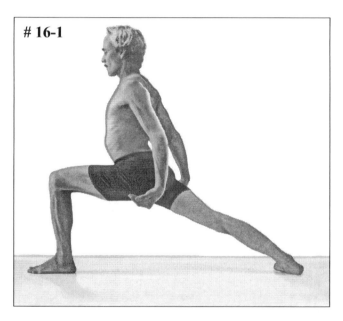

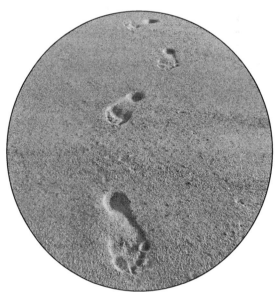

The journey is everything; destination is only footprints....

In the sands of time -----**Doug Swenson**

CHAPTER 5

Learning the Asanas
And Growing Your Practice

The greatest practice is found within
Integrity of action, embracing a peaceful heart and clarity of mind

The Sadhana Vinyasa Yoga system is a holistic approach designed to affect every area of your body and mind, rewarding you with balance and a sense of inner peace. This program combines the best of both the challenging and soft form asana practice routines, embracing a melody of softness and strength, power and tranquility. This program encourages the use of proper yoga sequencing to avoid injury, create enhanced comfort and energy flow. In this chapter, you will find breathing techniques and yoga sequencing, with a list of yoga asana categories and finally the asana instructions with cautions and posture options.

Regardless of your level of practice, I suggest you begin by practicing the various yoga routines without the suggested connecting vinyasa links, until you gain some confidence, and feel comfortable in the different poses. After practicing a few routines… by all means embrace the vinyasa with your very soul and weave it into your regular practice. If you first gain a little self-confidence, then your flow will feel more comfortable, yet powerful and energizing as your yoga takes on the essence of the blissful softness and incredible strength of nature.

Yoga Breathing vs. Traditional Yoga Breathing

While all forms of yoga breathing are similar, each has its own subtle yet important differences. In traditional soft-style yoga, many teachers use a similar *ujjayi* breathing technique you have just learned in this section, although in some traditional Yoga breathing, you are often taught to expand the lower abdominal muscles on inhalations and contract the lower abdominal muscles on the exhalation. In Sadhana Vinyasa Yoga, you will keep these muscles firm in order to assist in creating core strength and control.

If you rush your yoga practice, the breath is often a bit rushed too, which can lead to a loss of potential energy and sacrifice the tranquil yoga flow. For best results, you are encouraged to adapt a continuous slow, deep breathing rhythm to enhance energy, as well as creating inner calm and focus. This simple basic rule will assist your yoga asana practice, enhance your lung capacity, and build a strong foundation for all aspects of a successful yoga practice.

Philosophy of Practice

Sadhana Vinyasa Yoga teaches yoga practice as a priceless gift, a luxury with potential to positively affect every aspect of your whole life in a positive way. You can do anything as long as you believe in yourself; yoga can give you the confidence and energy to succeed.

At the same time success should not be measured in money, material goods, or popularity. In yoga practice and life, we base success on how we live our lives, how we influence and affect others and this planet, with a sense of gratitude. The best gift you can acquire is awareness the best gift you can give is love and kindness.

Yoga Sequencing

When creating a yoga routine, the aspect of yoga sequencing should not be overlooked, or you will risk injury, lose energy, and disrupt the flow. In the categories listed below, I have arranged the categories in an outline of suggested proper yoga sequence. If you are creating your own routine, simply start at the first category and progress toward the end, picking one or two postures from each category. There are other formats for building a balanced routine, yet this one is one of my favorites and creates a nice energy, without risking cumulative injury.

The Asana Practice

In this chapter, you will find the yoga asanas I have used to build the various different yoga routines. The actual yoga routines prescribed for the different levels of practice you will find in **(Chapters 6, 7, and 8)**. Also, it is important for you to make sure you review **(Chapter 2)**, to fully embrace the proper preparations and approach to this unique yoga practice and to understand the foundational concepts.

Navigating the Asana

In order to provide you with easy navigation and clarity, you will find, I have divided the traditional yoga postures *(asanas)*, into ten different sub-categories.

1 - Warm-ups & Cool Down

2 - Seated Poses

3 - Cat Stretch / Sun Salutations

4 - Standing Postures

5 - Headstand / Shoulder Stand (Inversions)

6 - Leg Stretches

7 - Back Stretches

8 - Spinal Twist

9 - Arm Balancing

10 - Deep Relaxation

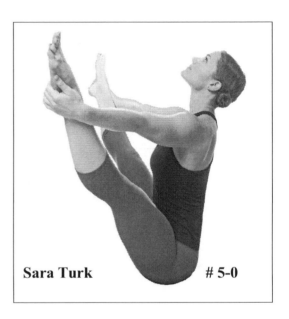

Sara Turk   # 5-0

THE TEN CATEGORIES OF YOGA ASANA PRACTICE

For the purpose of organization and easy access, I have divided the yoga asana practice into ten separate categories. These categories will make it easy for you to understand and practice your own yoga, and help you to teach balanced routines, or build your own routines.

1. **Yoga Warm-ups / Cool-downs:** Every yoga routine should begin with some gentle, yet active movements to prepare the body and mind for practice. At the beginning of a routine, this will increase your circulation, warm your muscles, and at the same time give you a connection with gentle, flowing movement. Warm-ups are usually less traditional exercises and can come in many forms, which can represent versions of traditional asana.

Cool-down Exercises: These are at the end of your practice and designed to gradually slow the heart, cool and calm the body and remove any tension created from a challenging asana practice. Cool down exercises are often the same warm-ups, practiced with a different motive, and you may use creatively- at your own discretion.

2. **Seated Postures:** These are some of the most fundamental aspects of yoga practice. They give you a good base for practicing breathing exercises, meditation, and act as a transition for moving into, or out of a practice routine. Just as yoga breathing isn't the same as normal breathing, sitting during yoga isn't the same old thing you do every day. You don't want to just dash into the seated poses like a winner on a television game show. In order to get the most from your whole routine, you need to enter the seated postures slowly, embracing correct body alignment and breathing techniques.

3. **Cat Stretch / Sun Salutations:** These are both active exercises, but the Sun Salutation, is traditionally an honoring of the sun, to be practiced at sunrise, or sunset, the two most tranquil times of day. In format, the salutations can be further divided into (two sub-categories), soft and hard — each representing a balance of various traditional yoga asanas mindfully woven together, with a vinyasa, or connecting link.

4. **Standing Postures:** Standing postures are yoga postures which are achieved by practicing asanas standing on one or both feet. Standing poses will stretch and strengthen your legs and torso creating better balance and self-confidence. The standing postures are great for a whole body warm-up at the beginning of a routine, or as a cool down at the back of a routine.

5. **Headstand and Shoulder Stand (Inversions):** I have given Headstand and Shoulder Stand their own category because they are greatly beneficial and very unique. These two inverted postures will have positive benefits on many aspects of your anatomy creating a passive and calm state of mind, yet leaving you very refreshed and rejuvenated. If you spend a few minutes each day with inverted postures it is a welcome counter measure after spending hours upright and on your feet, with work and daily activities.

Caution with Inversions:

There are certain conditions in which inverted postures should be modified, or avoided altogether

1. If you are pregnant,
2. If you have glaucoma,
3. If you have severe injury to your neck,
4. If you have extreme high blood pressure,
5. If you have a floating retina, (eye injury)
6. If you are in your moon cycle — the choice is yours

6. **Leg Stretches:** Leg stretch postures lengthen and tone your leg muscles, joints, and tendons. These postures will create more pliable muscles, release stress, and tension, and help to prepare you for many other postures.

7. **Back Bending Postures:** Back bending postures are yoga postures which focus on arching your back. They lengthen, tone, and stretch your spine. These postures will create a more pliable spine and help to assist in proper vertebrae alignment. In addition, these postures help to expand your chest, correct round shoulders and strengthen back muscles. Keep your back healthy and strong through regular moderate yoga exercise and you will be active throughout your life.

8. **Twisting Postures:** Twisting postures are yoga postures which focus on your spine and back muscles by twisting, toning, and stretching your spine. These postures will create a more pliable spine and help to assist in proper vertebrae alignment. In addition, these postures help to overcome back aches and create more mobility of your spine and whole torso.

9. **Arm Balance Postures:** Arm Balance postures are yoga postures which focus on strengthening your arms, shoulders, and upper body. These postures also create self-confidence, enhance balance, and teach the philosophy of "softness as power." Arm balance postures will create muscle strength and toning by lifting your own body weight.

Generally speaking, the arm balance poses tend to be easier for intermediate to advanced students - although beginners should still give them a try to build foundation.

10. **Deep Relaxation Techniques and Postures:** The Corpse Pose coupled with the ancient technique of deep relaxation is traditionally used at the end of your yoga practice. This is designed to embrace a very relaxing element where you can foster peace, positive thinking and an overwhelming sensation of inner peace (Symbolically being re-born).

Counter Stretching: Counter Stretching **is not a category** it only refers to the practice of complementing one posture or a series of postures with another stretch, or asana, which will assist in relieving any tension from the previous pose. For example, if you completed a back bend and find tension in your back, you could add a counter stretch such as a Seated Forward Bend, or Supine Twist to release the tension and return your body to a neutral state. The counter stretches, I have suggested in this program are helpful to create balance, although you can also use your own best judgment.

CATEGORY 1 – WARM-UPS / COOL-DOWNS   (PG 77 – 85)

Cat 1 / # 1 - Neck Rolls:

Neck rolls are exactly what their name implies. In this exercise you will gently roll and stretch your neck. Make sure to move slowly and practice your yoga breathing throughout the exercise.

Benefits:

Neck rolls serve to warm up the muscles of your neck, release tension, and create flexibility as they lubricate the neck joint.

Caution:

*   Injury to Neck (be conscious)

Instructions: Neck Rolls - Cat 1 / # 1 (Pg 77 - 78)

1. Start by tilting your head slowly, moving gently forward and backward. Now tilt your head slowly from right to left side keeping your vision forward, as if you were going to touch your ear to your shoulder. Exhale as you tilt your head slowly to the right side, and then inhale back to center and exhale to the left side – inhale and return to center.

2. Now turn your head to the right, looking over your right shoulder. Return to facing forward, and repeat by turning your head to the left, looking back over your left shoulder. Repeat this left and right motion two times.

3. Proceed to roll your neck slowly and gently in a circular motion first to the right a two times, and then back to the left two times.

Cat 1 / # 2 - Shoulder Rolls:

Shoulders rolls get their name from the rolling motion of your shoulders. Make sure to move slowly and practice your yoga breathing throughout the exercise.

Benefits: Shoulder Rolls serve to warm up the muscles of your shoulders and upper back, release tension, and create a bit of flexibility.

Instructions: Shoulder Rolls - Cat 1 / # 2 (Pg 78)

1. Start by lifting your shoulders up by your ears on an inhale, and then exhale to rotate your shoulders back behind your back. Complete the circle by lowering your shoulders downward and then forward.

2. Strive to make this exercise flow in a circular motion, first in one direction for a few repetitions, then change directions and roll your shoulders back in the other direction.

Cat 1 / # 3 - Rocking Your Baby:

Doing this exercise, you look like a parent gently rocking a baby from side to side to sooth and calm the baby's spirit.

Benefits:

Rocking The Baby will open your hips and create more flexibility in your knees and ankles.

Cautions: Knee injury, lower back tension or neck injury.

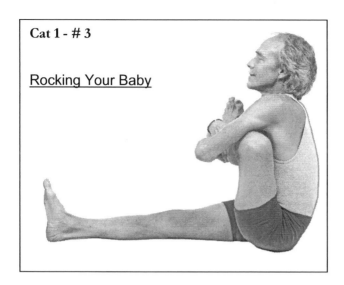

Cat 1 - # 3

Rocking Your Baby

Instructions: **Rocking Your Baby - Cat 1 / # 3 (Pg 79)**

1. Start in Seated Angle Pose **(Pg 87, # 2-A).** Bend your left knee and cradle your leg with your arms, pulling it into your chest like you are holding a baby. Hold this position and start your slow deep breathing **(photo # 3).**

2. Rock your bent leg from right to left with a gentle smooth motion as you continue your slow deep breathing, practice three or four repetitions **(photo # 3).**

3. On an exhalation pull your left bent leg, in toward your chest, up as high toward your shoulders as possible, releasing tension on exhalations and hold for a few breaths. When finished, lower your leg back to the floor and repeat steps 1–4 with the right leg.

Cat 1 / # 4 - Rock and Roll:

Rock and rolls are exactly what their name implies. In this exercise you will gently roll forward and backward on the floor.

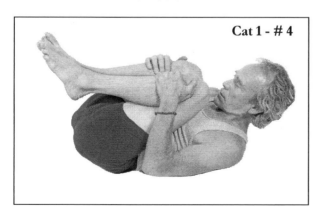

Cat 1 - # 4

Benefits:

Warm up the back muscles and spine, release tension, and create warmth on the back.

Caution:

- Back Injury
- Knee and Hip injury

Instructions: <u>**Rock and Rolls - Cat 1 / # 4 (Pg 79 - 80)**</u>

1. Start by sitting on the floor - on a yoga mat or soft pad, hug your knees and get ready to roll forward and backward, being mindful not to hurt your neck, or back **(photo 4).**

2. Try 4-5 repetitions then relax on your back for a few moments.

Cat 1 / # 5 - Chi Stretch:

The Chi Stretch is similar to exercises in Thai Chi, not just stretching — yet a moving meditation and awareness of energy.

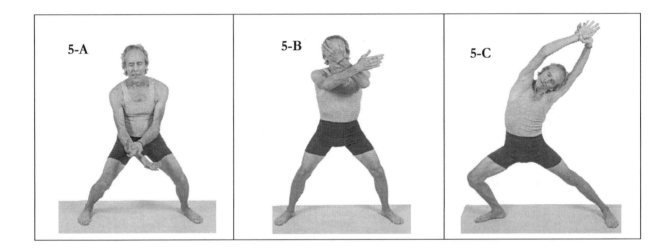

Benefits:

Warm up the legs, arms and torso and spine, release tension, and create awareness.

Caution:

- Back injury (Be conscious)
- Knee injury

Instructions: <u>**Chi Stretch - Cat 1 / # 5 (Pg 80 - 81)**</u>

1. Start in a wide standing position with hands by your sides. On an inhalation reach out wide with your arms, then in toward your body, bending your knees as you lift arms upward **(photo # 5-A).** Continue to raise your arms crossed up in front of your face **(photo # 5-B).**

2. Now open your arms, and begin to exhale as you grasp your right wrist, up over your head with your left hand, pulling your upper body to the left as you lunge to the right, bending your right knee **(photo # 5-C).**

3. Repeat this exercise on the opposite side; try 2 repetitions on each side.

Cat 1 / # 6 - Young Hips:

This young hip warm-up is a slow and relaxing exercise similar to practicing for salsa dance — as we try to slowly and gently lubricate the hip joints.

Benefits:

Warm up the hips, arms and lower torso as you gain flexibility in the spine.

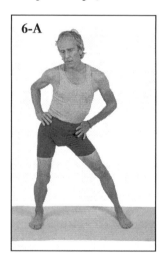
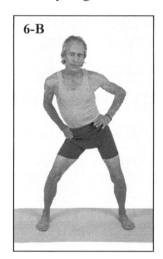

Caution:

- Fragile Hips (Be conscious)
- Hip replacement (Be aware)

Instructions: Young Hips - Cat 1 / # 6 (Pg 81)

1. Start in a wide standing position with hands on your hips; now gently rock your hips from right to left for 2 repetitions.

2. Then repeat in a circular motion for 2 additional repetitions **(photo # 6-A / 6-B).**

Cat 1 / # 7 - Pendulum (Front to Back):

In this exercise you will resemble a pendulum swinging free with fluid momentum.

Benefits:

Warm up the hips and legs, as you inspire coordination and balance.

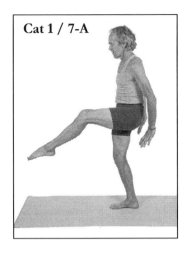

Cat 1 / 7-A

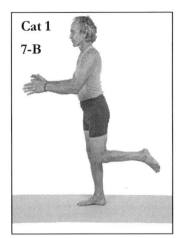

Cat 1
7-B

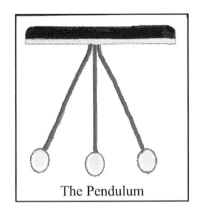

The Pendulum

Caution:

- Fragile Hips (Be conscious)
- Hip replacement (Be conscious)

Instructions: Pendulum (Front to Back) - Cat 1 / # 7 (Pg 81 - 82)

1. Start in a standing position with arms hanging free by your sides; now balance on your right leg as you swing your left leg forward and backward, at the same time allowing your arms to swing in the opposite direction as your leg. Repeat 2-3 times on each leg **(photo # 7-A & 7-B).**

Cat 1 / # 8 - Pendulum (Side to Side):

The same description, benefits and cautions apply to (this side to side pendulum) variation as with warm-up # 7, the front to back variation, only now with a different range of motion.

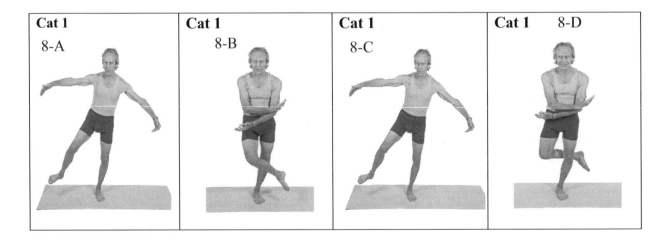

Cat 1
8-A

Cat 1
8-B

Cat 1
8-C

Cat 1   8-D

Instructions: Pendulum (Side to Side) - Cat 1 / # 8 (Pg 82 - 83)

1. Start in a standing position with arms hanging free by your sides, and feet about two feet apart. Now balance on your left leg as you swing your right leg to the right, at the same time allowing both arms to swing open with your leg **(photo # 8-A)**.

2. Then allow the right leg to swing back across the front of your left leg, at the same time crossing your arms in front of your torso **(photo # 8-B)**.

3. Now repeat, swinging leg to right again **(photo # 8-C)** only this time, when you swing back, bring right leg behind your left leg **(photo # 8-D)**. Repeat 2-3 times on each leg.

Cat 1 / # 9 - Sumo Stretch:

In this warm-up it has the flavor of a Sumo Wrestler warming up before a challenging match, yet it works well for yoga practice too.

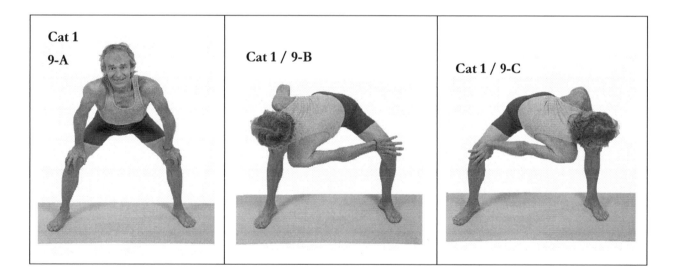

Benefits:

This is a great warm-up and stretch for the muscles of the back, shoulders and arms with an added tone-up of the spine. Creates warmth in the feet and inspires balance.

Caution:

Fragile Hips (Be conscious) / Hip replacement (Be conscious)

Instructions: Sumo Stretch - Cat 1 / # 9 (Pg 83 - 84)

1. Start in a standing position with arms hanging free by your sides, and feet about two feet apart. Now bend your knees and allow your hands to rest on top of each knee as you drop your weight evenly **(photo 9-A)**.

2. Take a slow deep inhalation and, as you exhale, twist your upper body to your right as you drop your left shoulder and exhale **(photo 9-B)**.

3. Now inhale back to back to position **(photo # 9-A)** then exhale as you now twist your upper body to your left and you drop your right shoulder **(photo 9-C)**. Practice 2-3 times on each side.

Cat 1 / # 10 - Standing Body Twisting:

This is a spinal and body twist practiced from a standing position. This exercise is an easy way to gradually warm your entire body for practice.

Benefits:

This exercise relieves tension along your spine and throughout your torso. It also creates some basic heat and flexibility needed to assist you in your yoga asanas.

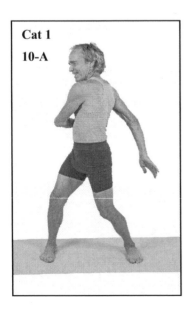

Cat 1
10-A

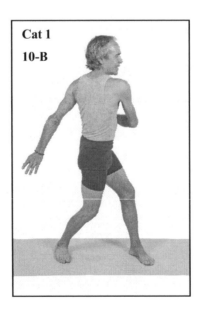

Cat 1
10-B

Cautions:
- Knee injury
- Hip injury
- Back injury

Instructions: <u>Standing Body Twisting - Cat 1 / # 10 (Pg 84 - 85)</u>

1. Stand with your feet a little more than shoulders-width apart. Twist and rotate your torso from right side **(photo # 10-A)** to your left side **(photo # 10-B)** in a slow, yet steady pace, allowing your arms to swing free as you move your body from right to left.

2. Practice two to four repetitions. When finished stand quietly and relax for a few breaths with your arms relaxed by your sides.

<u>**Cat 1 / # 11 - Wrist Exercises:**</u> These simple exercises are an excellent toner for the wrist and preventative medicine.

Benefits:

In this exercise you will create flexibility on the tops and bottoms of your wrists as you strengthen the bottom sides of your forearms. The tops of your wrists will become more pliable, and you will release tension and reduce the chance of injury.

Instructions: <u>Wrist Exercises - Cat 1 / # 11 (Pg 85)</u>

1. Clench your fists, palms facing upward, and keeping your lower arms stationary as you bend your wrists upward and downward 2-3 repetitions, then relax.

2. Clench your fists with palms facing downward, and keeping your lower arms stationary as you bend your wrists upward and downward 2-3 repetitions, then relax.

3. Clench your fists, knuckles facing each other, and keeping your lower arms stationary as you bend your wrists sideways, upward and downward 2-3 repetitions, then relax.

4. Clench your fists, and you rotate your wrists in a circular motion. First circle your wrists to the right, then change directions and circle your wrists back to the left.

~ When finished Shake your hands a bit and relax ~

(Always practice mindfully and use these exercise as preventative maintenance)

Cat 2 / # 1 - Jnana Mudra:

In Sanskrit, *jnana* means "knowledge" and a *mudra* is a "seal" or "lock." Often seated poses include specific placement of your hands and fingers. Traditionally, yogis use *jnana mudra* in many seated asana and as a focal point in meditation. In *jnana mudra*, your index finger represents your individual soul, and your thumb represents the universal soul. As you unite the tip of your thumb to the tip of your index finger, you symbolically unite the energy of your soul with the energy of the whole universe. The result of this unification is knowledge.

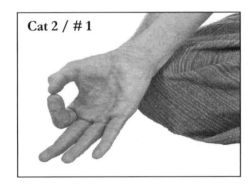

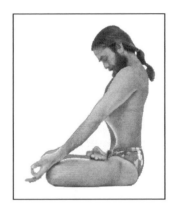

Benefits:

Energetically this mudra helps to recycle energy back into your body, creates focus and inner peace. At the same time joining the energy of the individual soul with the energy of the universe, allowing for the concept of – all things are possible.

Cautions:

- Cramping in the fingers, or hands

Instructions: <u>Jnana Mudra / Cat 2, # 1 (Pg 86)</u>

1. Sit on the floor in Perfect Posture **(Pg 88 / # 3),** or any of your favorite seated postures listed in this section).

2. Place your hands on your knees with your palms facing upward.

3. Open your hands and touch your index finger to the tip of your thumb. Your remaining fingers should be straight, but not stiff or tense **(photo # 1).**

Cat 2 / # 2 - Seated Angle Pose:

In this relaxing pose, you will form a 90-degree angle with your legs and torso.

Benefits:

The Seated Angle Pose corrects your posture, strengthens the muscles of your back, and opens the energy flow in your chest. Many people who have trouble with their knees will find the Seated Angle a good alternative to the cross-legged seated poses.

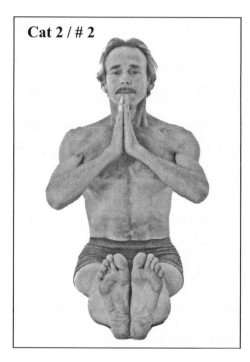

Cat 2 / # 2

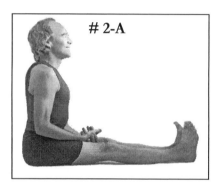

2-A

Cautions:

- Lower Back Tension
- Tightness in Neck
- Shoulder injury

Vinyasa: (Hard - Vin # 2 / Soft - Vin # 4, 6, or 7)

Instructions: Seated Angle / Cat 2 / # 2 (Pg 87)

1. Sit on the floor with both legs extended out in front, your spine straight, and your shoulders back.

2. Keep your feet pointing upward and slightly flexed, as you fold your hands in your lap, or over your heart **(photo # 2 / 2-A)**. If your lower back is rounded, try placing a small pillow under your knees: this can help nudge your body into the proper posture. Hold this position for five to ten slow, deep breaths.

Cat 2 / # 3 - Perfect Posture (*Siddhasana*):

In Sanskrit, *siddha* means "perfect." A *siddha* is also a great "prophet" or a "sage", one who is very pure and spiritual. As you practice this Perfect Posture, you're connecting with the wisdom of the ancient Yoga masters.

Benefits:

Perfect Posture promotes flexibility in your knees, ankles, and thighs, and it also contributes to attaining excellent posture. Many cultures use the position in everyday life as a way to relax, and meditate, socialize and to take a moment to reflect on gratitude of simplicity.

History:

This asana is actually like using training wheels on a bicycle, as the simple pose will train you to achieve many other yoga asanas such as the following: Half Lotus Pose, Full Lotus Pose, and many other asanas where flexibility of the knees, ankles, and hips are in use. At the same time, this asana teaches you good posture, a simple way to ground out, and find closeness to the Earth.

For some of us this asana can be quite challenging, due to body types, lifestyle or past injury and yet with regular mindful practice, comfort will be found.

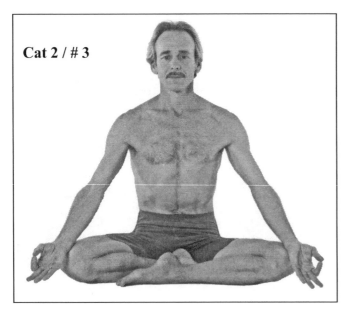

Cat 2 / # 3

Cautions:

- Knee Joint Stress
- Lower Back Tension
- Tightness in Neck

Modifications:

Sit on a blanket and place pillows or blocks under your knees.

Instructions: <u>Perfect Posture - Cat 2 / # 3 (Pg 88 - 89)</u>

1. Start by sitting on the floor with your legs extended out in front of you, with your spine straight and your shoulders back.

2. Bend your right knee, grabbing your right ankle with your hands and pulling your foot in toward your groin. Now grab your left ankle and pull your left foot in toward your groin, placing your left foot to rest on the outside of your right ankle.

3. Now you are sitting cross-legged on the floor with your spine straight and your shoulders back **(photo # 3).** If you find this uncomfortable, place a small pillow under each knee. In addition, you might choose to place a small pillow under your hips in order to help correct your posture. For beginners, as an alternative you could sit on the edge of a large pillow with your feet on the floor, - keeping your back straight. More flexible students can lower their knees to the floor.

4. Extend your arms and rest your wrists and hands on your knees, with palms facing upward. Now place your fingers in the traditional *jnana mudra* position. Hold this position for five to ten slow, deep yoga breaths, remembering to close your eyes, calm your mind, and relax.

Cat 2 / # 4 - Full Lotus (*Padmasana*):

The word *padma* means "lotus." In this posture, you float like a water lily as you create the beauty of a lotus flower with your body and your mind. This is a very advanced pose, so be extremely gentle with your knees in the Lotus posture, and take your time in arriving at this pose.

Benefits:

This pose helps invigorate the nerves in your legs and thighs. It also helps loosen your knee joints and increases flexibility in your ankles and opens hips.

Cautions:

- Knee Joint Stress, Tightness in Neck and
- Lower Back Tension

Modifications:

Try sitting on a small blanket and then just place one leg in (½ lotus) with a pillow to support under the knee, or just practice perfect posture for an option.

> ➢ **Practice lotus right leg up first in one practice and left leg up first the next time.**

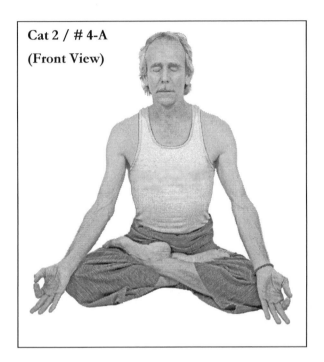

Cat 2 / # 4-A
(Front View)

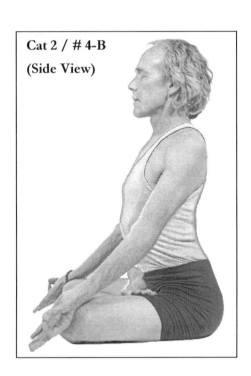

Cat 2 / # 4-B
(Side View)

Instructions: Full Lotus - Cat 2 / # 4 (Pg 89 - 91)

1. Sit on the floor in Easy Posture **(photo # 3)** with your back straight and your mind calm.

2. Take your right foot in your hands and slowly place it on your left thigh.

3. Take your left foot in your hands and slowly place it on your right thigh.

4. Be aware of correct posture as you open your chest and gently pull your shoulders back. Feel yourself relax as you sit proud with your chin held high.

5. Extend your arms over your thighs and rest your hands and wrists on your knees, with palms facing upward.

6. Place your hands in the *jnana mudra* position. You now are in the Full Lotus position **(photo # 4-A, 4-B).**

7. Close your eyes and hold this pose from five to ten slow deep breaths, calm the mind and relax, as you feel yourself gently floating.

8. When you are finished slowly take your feet out of lotus, to avoid injury.

9. In order to keep a balance of stretch in Lotus Posture, alternately placing your right foot up on your left thigh first, then the next time using your left foot up first.

Cat 2 / # 5 - Bound Lotus (*Baddha Padmasana*):

The word *baddha* means "caught" or "restrained" and *padmasana* is the "lotus posture." In this posture you will restrain your feet with your hands and arms.

Benefits:

In this posture you will receive the same benefits as the Lotus, plus an extra stretch through your arms, shoulders, and chest. You will find additional stretch to wrist and ankles.

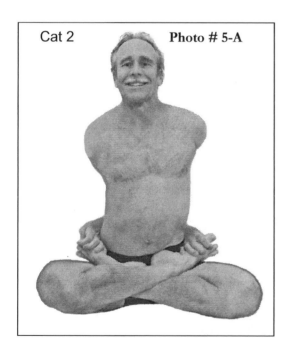

Cat 2   Photo # 5-A

Cautions:

- Knee Joint Stress
- Lower Back Tension
- Tightness in Neck
- Injury to Rotator Cup or Shoulders

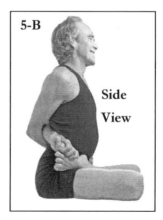

5-B

Side View

Modifications:

Hold a strap in both hands and behind your back to extend your reach, or just practice lotus, or perfect posture.

Instructions: Bound Lotus - Cat 2 / # 5 (Pg 91 - 92)

1. From the Full Lotus posture, reach behind your back with your left hand, and grab the toes of your left foot. If necessary, lean forward until you can take hold of your toes.

2. Repeat this process to reach behind your back with your right hand to grab toes of your right foot.

3. Sit up gradually, maintaining correct posture **(photo # 5-A, 5-B).** Hold this posture for 5 to 15 slow deep breaths.

4. When finished, release the grip of your hands on your toes. Take your feet out of lotus slowly, then gently stretch and shake out your legs and feet for a few moments.

Cat 2 / # 6 - Thunderbolt (*Vajrasana*):

The Sanskrit word *vajra* means "thunderbolt," but you sometimes see this same posture under the name Hero or Champion. This pose is a good alternative for the cross-legged poses, and it's a common base posture for meditation.

Benefits:

Thunderbolt stimulates nerves in your feet and lower legs, stretches muscles in your feet, and ankles. This pose helps to correct flat feet and promote better arches.

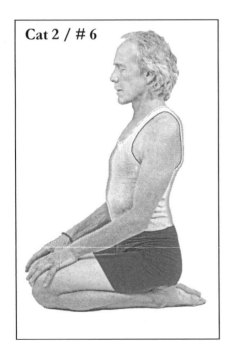

Cat 2 / # 6

Cautions:

- Knee Joint Stress
- Lower Back Tension
- Tightness in Neck
- Injury to Ankles

Modifications:

Separate the knees wider and rest the torso on a pillow or bolster.

Instructions: <u>Thunderbolt - Cat 2 / # 6 (Pg 92 – 93)</u>

1. Kneel on the floor, keeping your spine straight and shoulders back.

2. Sit back on your heels with your toes pointed backward. Feel your neck lengthen, and then fold your hands into your lap. If you have knee problems place a folded towel or small pillow between your calves and thighs, under your sit bones.

3. Place your gaze forward, parallel to the floor. Hold this position for 5 to 10 complete breaths **(photo # 6).**

<u>Cat 2 / # 7 - Cobbler (*Baddha Konasana*):</u>

In Sanskrit *baddha* means "caught" or "restrained" and *kona* means "angle," in this asana, you will hold onto the angles created with the bent knees, looking like a cobbler.

Benefits:

The Cobbler Pose is an excellent hip opener, also bringing flexibility to the ankles and inner thighs at the same time giving a stretch to the lower back.

Cautions: (Ankle Joint Stress, Lower Back Tension, Knee injury or hip injury).

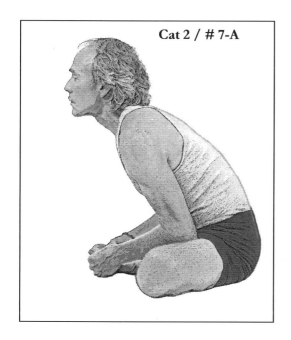

Cat 2 / # 7-A

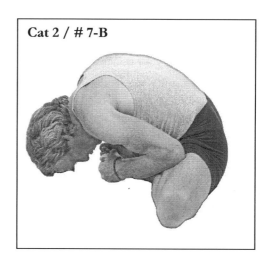

Cat 2 / # 7-B

Instructions: Cobbler - Cat 2 / # 7 (Pg 93 – 94)

1. Start by Siting in Seated Angle Pose **(Pg 87, # 2-A),** then bend your knees and try to move feet closer to your torso. Try to sit up straight as you prepare for the asana for a few breaths, then exhale as you slowly bend forward at the waist, extending your torso out over your bent knees, with elbow pushing on inner thighs **(photo # 7-A).**

2. Now pull your heels toward your pelvis, then drop your knees out to the sides toward the floor and press the soles of your feet together, or turned upward. Hold for 5 complete breaths **(photo # 7-B),** then exit slowly and mindfully.

Modifications: Sit on a small blanket or block and then place a block or pillow under both knees and maybe a bolster, or large pillow under your torso.

Cat 2 / # 8 – Child's Pose (*Balasana*):

Balasana translates as meaning Child's Pose and in this posture you will resemble a child resting for a nap after playing all day.

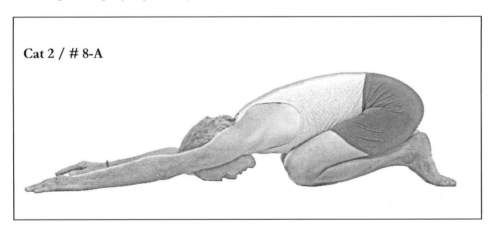

Cat 2 / # 8-A

Benefits:

Child's pose gently calms the body and mind as it stimulates the third eye point. Child's pose will stretch the low back and tones abdominal organs, as it stimulates digestion and elimination.

Modifications:

Place a blanket or pillow under hips, knees or head. If pregnant, spread the knees wide apart to remove any pressure on the abdomen. You may also need a folded towel under ankles.

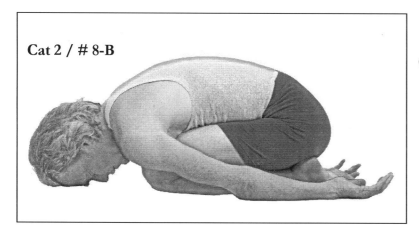

Cat 2 / # 8-B

Cautions:

- Weak or injured knees
- Stiff ankles

Instructions: <u>Child's Pose - Cat 2 / # 8 (Pg 94 – 95)</u>

1. Resting on hands and knees lower your hips to the heels and forehead to the floor. Have the knees together or if more comfortable, spread the knees slightly apart.
2. Place arms overhead with the palms on the floor **(photo # 8-A)** or the arms can be resting alongside the body with the palms facing upward **(photo # 8-B).**
3. Breathe slowly and deeply, holding for 5-6 breaths, or much longer.

Cat 2 / # 9 - Cow Face (*Gomukhasana*):

The word *gomukhanasa* translates as meaning "cows face pose" and in this asana you will be relaxed and easy, like a contented cow grazing in green grass.

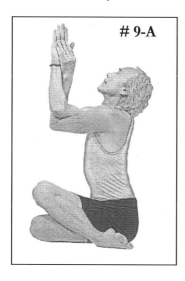
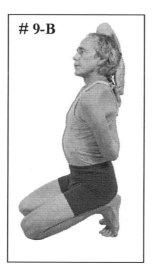
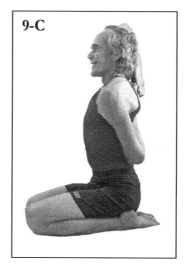

9-A   # 9-B   9-C

Benefits:

Cow Face Pose stretches shoulders and upper back, inspiring hips and ankles to gently open as it teaches inner focus.

Cautions:

Weak or injured knees and stiff ankles

Modifications:

Try sitting a small block or folded blanket to release tension from hips, ankles and knees.

Instructions: Cow Face - Cat 2 / # 9 (Pg 95 – 96)

1. Sit on the floor in a kneeling position, then using your hands lift your hips, try to cross the right leg over and on top of the left thigh, and walk both ankles out to the side of the hips.

2. Now inhale as you lift your arms up over your chest, resting your right bent elbow on top of your left bent elbow as you wrap one arm around the other arm **(photo # 9-A).**

3. Breathe deeply and hold 3-5 breaths, then gently come out of the pose and repeat the same asana only this this time crossing left leg on top and left arm on top for an additional 3-5 breaths.

4. **Variations: (photo # 9-B)** - Reach right hand over your right shoulder and left hand behind the middle back to grasp right hand behind your back. You may use a strap to extend reach. Try a different foot and ankle placement in **(photo # 9-C).**

Cat 2 / # 10 - Gracious Pose (_Bhadrasana_):

Bhadra in Sanskrit means "auspicious" or "gracious." This asana is simple and easy to perform, and often called: "**Seated Frog Pose,**" as it looks like a frog seated on the shore of a pond.

Benefits:

Gracious pose actively stretches the quadriceps, opens the hips, lengthens the spine, and promotes connection to earth and inner calm.

Traditional Meditation Pose:

This pose has often been used as a meditation posture, while seated on a cushion.

Modifications:

Sit on a small block, or folded blanket and pull knees closer together.

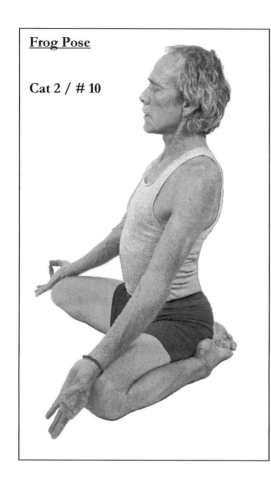

Frog Pose

Cat 2 / # 10

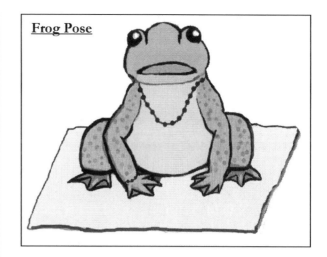

Frog Pose

Cautions:

Back injury, Hip injury, stiff Ankles

and Knee injury

There are 3-4 different variations of the Frog pose and yet each is a different pose in itself. The one thing in common is hip opening.

Instructions: Gracious Pose - Cat 2 / # 10 (Pg 96 – 97)

1. Begin by kneeling on the floor in Thunderbolt **(photo # 6, Pg 92)**. Then bring the knees (hips width apart) and ideally the big toes touching behind you. Carefully sit back on your heels with the heels touching the outside of your hips. Spread your knees as wide as comfortable. Rest the hands on the knees with the palms in *jnana mudra*, or palms facing down on top of your knees.

2. Lean back to the hips, and settle down into the floor. Then reach the crown of the head up to lengthen the spine. Drop the shoulders down and back, and move chest towards the front of the room **(photo # 10)**.

3. Hold for 5-7 complete breaths or as long as comfortable.

4. Afterward gently move your legs a bit to bring back the circulation and lessen the chance of knee injury.

Cat 2 / # 11 - Rabbit (*Sasangasana*):

Sasangasana translates as meaning "rabbit pose," due to the placement of your feet and torso which resemble a rabbit.

Benefits:

The Rabbit pose will lengthen the spine and stretch the back, arms, and shoulders while stimulating the immune and endocrine systems.

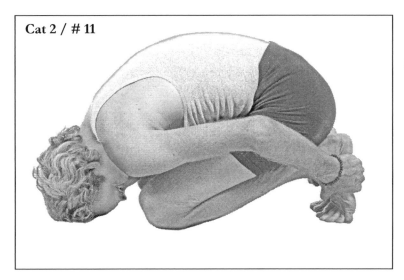

Cat 2 / # 11

Cautions:

- Weak or injured Knees
- Stiff Ankles, calf muscles

Modifications:

Place a folded blanket under the shin bones, ankles or knees and another under the head to protect them from pressure and stress.

Instructions: Rabbit Pose - Cat 2 / # 11 (Pg 98)

1. Start in the Child's Pose **(Pg 95, # 8-B)**, then flex feet, holding onto the heels with hands gently pulling your forehead close to knees with the top of the head on the floor.
2. If this is uncomfortable, place a folded blanket under your forehead and your knees, with a rolled towel under your shin bones. Arch your back upward and relax.
3. Breathe slowly and hold this position for 4-8 breaths **(photo # 11)**.
4. To release… slowly exhale and lower the hips to the heels and slide the forehead back to the floor into Child's pose.

Cat 2 / # 12 - Boat Pose (*Navasana*):

The Sanskrit name *nava,* translates as meaning "boat or ship," and in this pose you resemble a boat floating in the water.

Benefits:

In the Boat Pose, you strengthen the muscles of your stomach, legs, and arms. This posture helps firm your waistline and tone your kidneys while you develop strength and power.

Vinyasa:

Hard – (Vin # 2) - **Pg 53**

Soft – (Vin # 5, 6, or 7) – **Pg 57 – 59**

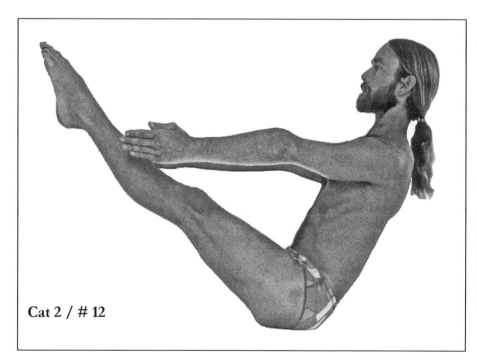

Cat 2 / # 12

Cautions:

- Back injury
- Neck injury
- Pregnancy

Modifications:

Keep your knees slightly bent, or practice with one leg bent and resting one foot on the floor. Sit on towel for comfort.

Instructions: Boat Pose - Cat 2 / # 12 (Pg 99 – 100)

1. Start in the Seated Angle Pose **(Pg 87, # 2-A).** Then bend your knees, and lift your feet up off the floor, as you balance on your buttocks, with arms extended out parallel to the ground. **To Modify:** you may choose to sit on a folded towel, or keep knees bent.

2. Now try to straighten your legs and form a strong core pose, as you balance in this position for 3-5 breaths **(photo # 12)**.

3. When finished exhale, lowering your legs to the floor, and relax into the Seated Angle Posture, or move through your next vinyasa.

Cat 2 / # 13 - Staff Pose (*Dandasana*):

Danda means a "staff" or "rod." In this posture your arms on either side of your hips will resemble a staff or rod supporting your torso.

Benefits:

In the Staff Pose, you will expand your chest, stretch the backside of your neck, enhancing posture and expanding lung capacity. This is a great position to help overcome bad posture and is used as a base to flow into other postures.

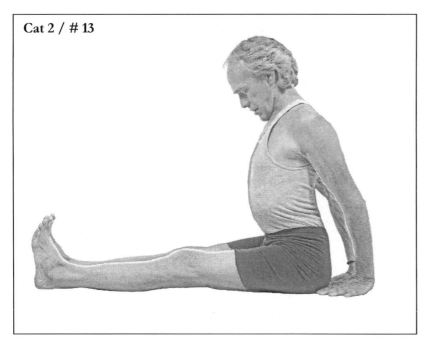

Cat 2 / # 13

Cautions:

- Wrist problems
- Back injury
- Stiff neck

Modifications:

Place a folded blanket under the hips, or a small pillow under the knees. If you have short arms place a slight elevation under your hands.

Vinyasa:

Hard: (Vin # 2) - **Pg 53** / **Soft:** (Vin # 5, 6, or 7) – **Pg 57 - 59**

Instructions: Staff Pose - Cat 2 / # 13 (Pg 100 – 101)

1. Start from the Seated Angle position **(Pg 87, # 2-A).** Place your hands on the floor, outside of your hips and slightly behind you – if possible.

2. Palms facing downward and your fingers pointing forward toward your toes. Drop your head forward into your chest, like you were trying to look down at your navel.

3. Pull your shoulders backward and downward. Really expand your chest, exaggerating it, push your chest way out as you arch your back. Flex your feet upward, close your eyes and start doing your slow deep breathing for five deep breaths **(photo # 13).** When finished, inhale and then move though a vinyasa to the next pose.

Cat 2 / # 14 - Garland Pose (*Malasana*):

In Sanskrit the word *mala* means "garland" and *asana* means "pose" or "seat." In India, garlands of flowers or beads are often used as ritual offerings and altar decoration. Traditionally, this hip opening pose was to prepare for seated position in meditation.

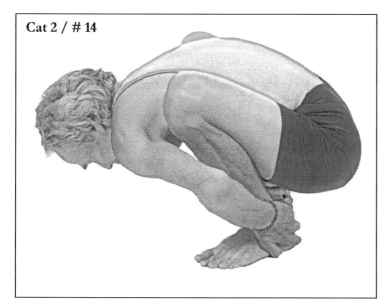

Cat 2 / # 14

Cautions:

- Back injury
- Knee injury
- Angle injury

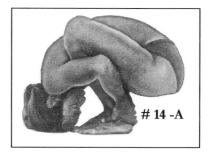

14 -A

Benefits:

The Garland Pose stretches the thighs, hips, groin, ankles, and torso. It also tones the abdominal muscles and helps to improve the function of the colon to help with elimination. Many have found this asana to improve balance, concentration, and focus, along with being particularly beneficial for women who are pregnant, as it can later aid in childbirth.

Modifications:

If your heels don't come to the floor, place a yoga wedge, folded blanket or rolled yoga mat underneath your heels. Some students will find sitting on a yoga block helpful, or try this pose with your back against a wall.

Vinyasa: <u>Hard:</u> (Vin # 2) - **Pg 53** / **Soft**: (Vin # 4, 5, 6, or 7) – **Pg 55 - 59**

Instructions: <u>Garland Pose - Cat 2 / # 14 (Pg 101 – 102)</u>

1. Start this asana in Mountain Pose **(Pg 136, photo # 14),** with your arms at your sides and feet about as wide as your mat.

2. Now bend your knees and slowly lower your hips, coming into a squatting position. Separate your thighs so they are slightly wider than your torso and try to keep your feet flat with heels down, if possible.

3. Move your torso slightly forward between knees and bring your upper arms and elbows to the outside of your knees. Pressing your elbows along the outside of your legs. **Beginners:** stay more upright with your palms together in prayer position.

4. **Intermediate to Advanced**: work toward dropping the head down toward the ankles and grasping the heels with your hands **(Pg 101, photo # 14 and 14-A).**

5. Hold for five breaths, then release slowly and relax into a crossed legged position, or move through a vinyasa.

6. **Options**: Experienced students may step their feet completely together, then move the torso between the legs, dropping the head down to the ankles and reaching both arms behind your back to clasp hands.

Cat 2 / # 15 - Happy Baby Pose (*Ananda Balasana*):

The word *ananda* means "happy" and *balasana* means "child" or "baby." In this asana you will feel youthful as you lay on you back and smile like a happy baby. This pose is not necessarily one of the traditional poses found in older hatha yoga texts, and yet is very popular in contemporary practice.

Benefits:

This asana gently stretches the inner groin and the back of the spine as it calms the brain and helps relieve stress and fatigue. Many students find this pose to be a great counter stretch for backbends, or forward bends, as it releases tensions from the back and massages the spine.

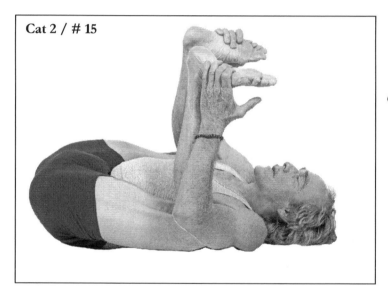

Cat 2 / # 15

Cautions:

- Pregnancy
- Knee injury
- Neck injury

Modifications:

Support your head and back on a blanket, and if you can't easily hold your feet with your hands, try using a yoga strap around the arch of your feet to extend reach.

Vinyasa: (Inhale to Cobra, or Up Dog Pose / Exhale to Child Pose, then to Happy Baby pose.

Instructions: Happy Baby Pose - Cat 2 / # 15 (Pg 103 – 104)

1. Start from Corpse Pose **(Pg 206, photo # 1),** laying on your back, and then bend your knees into your belly. Hold the outsides of your feet with your hands, opening your knees slightly wider than your torso and then bring knees up toward your armpits.

2. Gently push hands down on your feet, holding this position for 5 breathes **(photo 15)** then relax back into Corpse Pose.

3. **Options**: While holding your feet, gently rock from right to left side.

CATEGORY 3 – CAT & SUN SALUTATIONS   (PG 104 – 115)

The Cat Stretch and Sun Salutation are yoga exercises which are practiced in motion, as if one long vinyasa. In order to provide better assistance in this section you will be given many photos, with less, instructions which will give you a very visual understanding of the flow.

You will be given simple and yet very beneficial instructions:
   a) Background of the Cat Stretch and Sun Salutation
   b) Benefits and Cautions
   c) Modifications

Beyond that in the flow of asana there are 3 simple instructions:
   (1) – **In = Inhale -** (At this point in the flow it is best to Inhale)
   (2) – **Ex = Exhale -** (At this point in the flow it is best to Exhale)
   (3) – **Hold -** (This means to hold the asana for a duration - of breaths.

Example: (Hold – 5) is asking you to hold for 5 slow deep breaths.

   The Pace: (You may adjust the pace of movement to suit your own needs)

   a) **Quicker movements** create more heat, yet are less calming and create an active mind.
   b) **Slower movements** create less heat, yet instill a very soothing and peaceful inner calm.

Which is Correct - Quicker or Slower Pace?

Both concepts are correct and should be alternated over a period of practiced sessions in order to create balance and greater awareness.

> ➢ **The Cat Stretch Begins Here:**

Category # 3 - Cat Stretch (*Marjariasana*) # A

A - Cat Stretch:

When practicing this warm-up exercise you will resemble a cat stretching after a nice long nap. This warm-up movement can also be used as a subtle vinyasa for select postures.

Benefits:

The Cat Stretch tones, strengthens, and stretches your back muscles and can make your entire spine feel stronger and more flexible. Use awareness when it comes to props and do what works best for you, your body type, flexibility, strength, and motives for practice. This includes the use of a folded blanket under your knees, regulating room temperature and use of background music. In time, through these flowing yoga movements, as you embrace awareness of breath and being in the moment, you will become in sync with the concept of a moving meditation.

Options:

Placing a folded blanket under your knees is always helpful and comfortable option, which will help protect against cumulative injury, or especially if you have injury to the knees.

Suggestions:

Take your time with the Cat Stretch and always remember you can vary the repetitions and format. The Cat Stretch I have listed in this chapter is a basic version which will be most beneficial to the general population, although I still practice this simple exercise on many occasions and it is always delivers a very positive result. Other times I will hold parts of the exercise longer, or use a variety of moves, it is your practice.

Cat 3 / # A - Cat Stretch:

Practice 1-2 repetitions on each side, and then relax into Child's Pose **(Pg 94 - photo # 8-A).**

> **(In = Inhale / Ex = Exhale / Hold = Number of breaths)**

A-1 / Ex	A-2 / In	A-3 / Ex
A-4 / In	A-5 / EX	A-6 / In

> **Repeat the same sequence – on the opposite side and (practice 1 -2 repetitions).**

> **When finished rest in Child's Pose for 5 - 7 breaths.**

Cautions: Knee injury, back injury,

Hip injury and neck injury.

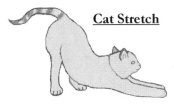

Cat Stretch

Instructions: Cat Stretch - Cat 3 / # A (Pg 105 – 107)

1. Start from a position resting on your hands and knees with torso parallel to the floor, then exhale all your air as you arch your back like a cat **(photo A-1).**

2. Now inhale and slowly drop your chest and shoulders toward the floor as you sway your back **(photo A-2).**

3. Then on an exhalation lift the torso, as you arch your back once again **(photo A-3).**

4. On our next inhalation lift your left leg back and up, as you arch your back, expand your chest and gaze upward **(photo A-4).**

5. On your next exhalation bring your left knee in toward your chest, trying to touch your knee to your nose **(photo A-5)**.

6. Now inhale and slowly drop your chest and shoulders toward the floor as you sway your back **(photo A-6)**. This completes one repetition.

Category # 3 - Sun Salutation (*Suryanamaskar*):

(In this section I list 3 different Sun Salutations – it is best to rotate your practice and try to embrace a variety of choices).

Sun Salutations (*Suryanamaskar*):

Since the dawn of Yoga practice there has been evidence of students practicing the Sun Salutation. The Sun Salutation is actually a combination of several different yoga postures connected together with a vinyasa, and serves as one of the best-known yoga warm-up exercises.

The Sanskrit word for Sun Salutation is *Suryanamaskar*. *Surya* means the "sun" and *Namaskar* means "blessing," "prayer" or "salutation." The Sun Salutation is very sacred and important Yoga exercise and is a healthy way to pay respect to the sun and at the same time salute the ultimate good within you.

Three Salutations (Easy or Challenging)

1. **Soothing Touch Salutation** is perfect for beginners, and takes a minimal amount of energy. Regardless of your level of practice you will find this basic Sun Salutation very tranquil, fun, and beneficial.

2. **Power Zone Salutation** works best for intermediate – advanced, with a short yet more challenging atmosphere

3. **Fluid Power Salutation** is a combination of longer duration and more challenging flow of asanas laced together to form a beautiful and yet challenging progression.

Benefits:

All Sun Salutations benefit most areas of your body. The stretching and counter-stretching of the torso rejuvenates your spine to help relieve back pain. The Sun Salutation stretches and strengthens your arm and leg muscles and promotes flexibility in your ankles, knees, and hip joints. The gentle, fluid transition from stretch to counter-stretch combined with yoga breathing techniques leaves your mind in a very tranquil, yet alert and focused state.

Salutation # 1

Category 3 / # 1 - Soothing Touch Salutation (Beg – Inter):

This is an easy, gentle, and relaxing salutation, based on a very traditional soft form practice with flavors of Integral and Sivananda yoga styles and is often referred to as the Moon Salutation, due to the cooler, softer, and more feminine aspects. You are welcome to use props, if it deems necessary. Take your time breathe deeply and strive to become a moving meditation.

Practice 2-4 repetitions then relax into mountain pose.
  ➤ (In = Inhale / Ex = Exhale / Hold = Number of breaths)

Cat 3 / # 1 - Soothing Touch Salutation (All Levels)   (Sequence 1-A to 1- X)

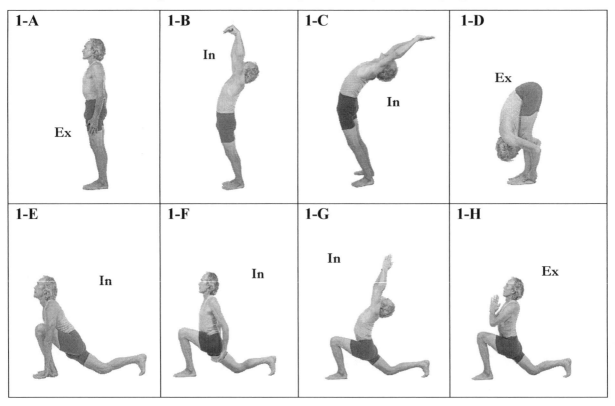

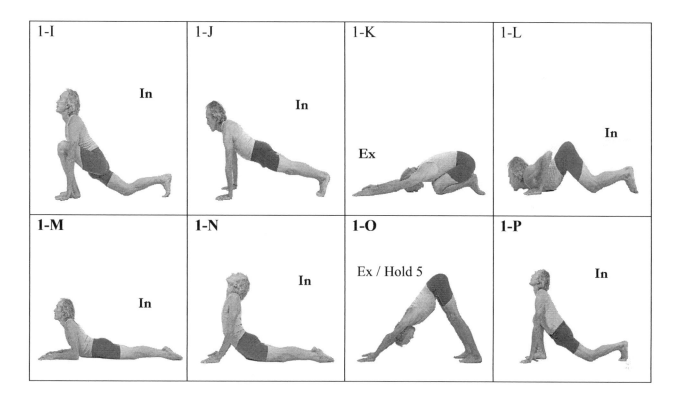

Important Note - In Photo **(1-S and 1-T)** you are still facing the same direction. The illustration is showing the back side to view arm placement.

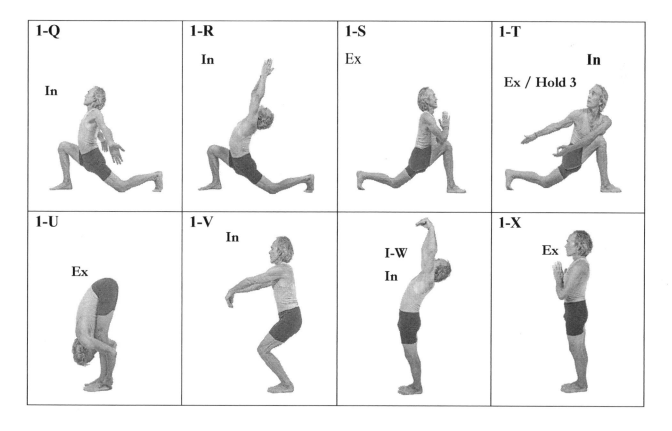

Sun Salutation # 2

Category 3 / # 2 - Power Zone Salutation (Inter - Adv):

This progression is derived from influences of the style of Ashtanga Yoga by K. Pattabhi Jois. The flavor of the flow is powerful, builds heat and self-confidence and is usually very challenging for most people. You may adjust the pace, although it is best to alternate with some days of slower pace and other times faster to create a balance.

Practice 2-5 repetitions then relax into Mountain Pose.
  ➤ (IN = Inhale / EX = Exhale / Hold = Number of breaths)

Cat 3 / # 2 – Power Zone Sun Salutation (All Levels) (Sequence 2-A to 2-M)

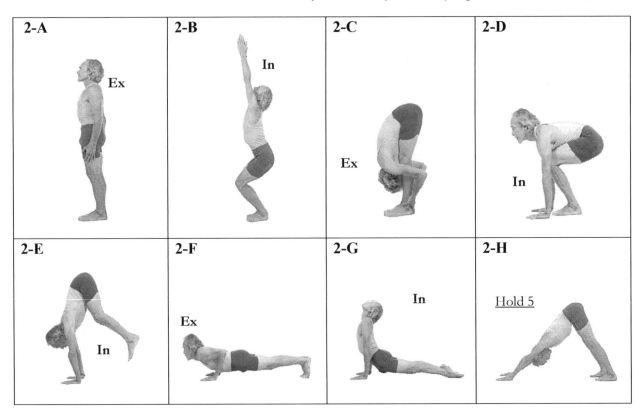

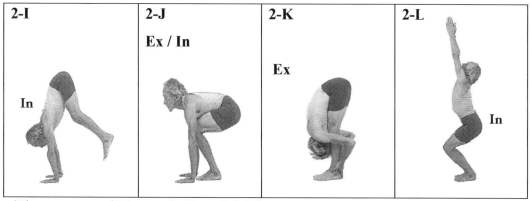

| 2-I | 2-J
Ex / In | 2-K

Ex | 2-L |

(Then return to / **Mountain Pose # 2-M**)

Practiced in (sets of two), Use your own best judgment -

You can do more or less – yet try to practice in sets of two.

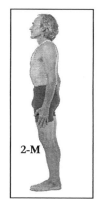

2-M

Sun Salutation # 3

Cat 3 / # 3 - Fluid Power Salutation (Inter – Adv):

If you want a more challenging energetic flow with your salutation, you can take on the **Fluid Power Salutation**. The Fluid Power Sun Salutation is very beautiful and can greatly help you to develop maximum strength and stamina along with inner peace of a moving meditation. After many years of practice, I was inspired to put this salutation together, using aspects of both hard and soft salutations, creating a very fluid and yet quite challenging flow.

Benefits:

The benefits are the same as the other Salutations – only with added power and strength, balance and muscle resistance along with a bit more cardio. One additional caution is to be aware of the wrist and take it easy.

This Sun Salutation is much longer than many traditional Sun Salutations, and with that in mind, please be mindful to take your time, remember to breathe slowly and practice with awareness.

Focus on embracing a beautiful flow from one pose to the next, instead of thinking of each separate asana – allow the energy of the parts to become one.

In time, you will weave through the energy of the different asana as a moving meditation. If you want to build strength you can pick one practice session and hold each separate frame, or part for 5 breaths and then on other sessions keep the flow and move a bit quicker.

Important Note –

In this sequence you will always face the same direction – the illustrations show the backside of some asana for vision of arm placement and body alignment.

Practice 2-5 repetitions then relax into Mountain Pose.

➤ (IN = Inhale / EX = Exhale / Hold = Number of breaths)

Cat 3 / # 3 – Fluid Power Sun Salutation (Inter - Adv)   (Sequence 1-A to 1- X)

3-1	3-2	3 / # 3 (Hold 3)	3 / # 4 Hold 3
Ex	In	Ex	In
3 / # 5	3 / # 6	3 / # 7	3 / # 8
Ex	In	Ex	In

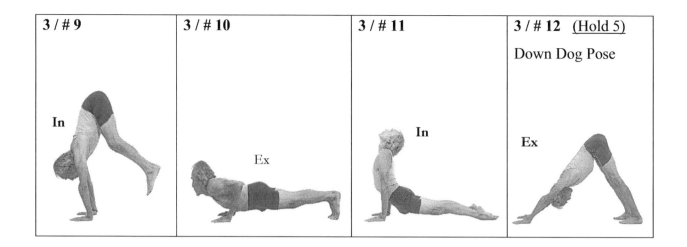

3 / # 9	3 / # 10	3 / # 11	3 / # 12 (Hold 5) Down Dog Pose
In	Ex	In	Ex

➢ Pose 3 - # 19 – is a Warrior II – as indicated

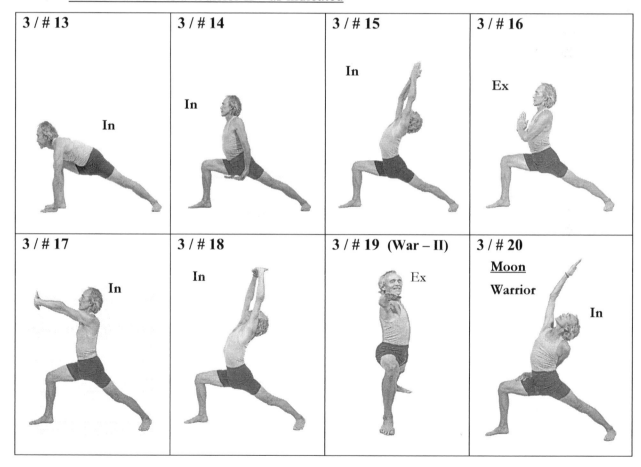

3 / # 13	3 / # 14	3 / # 15	3 / # 16
In	In	In	Ex
3 / # 17	3 / # 18	3 / # 19 (War – II)	3 / # 20 Moon Warrior
In	In	Ex	In

Try to move seamlessly from one asana to the next – being strong and yet powerful.

Continue this salutation on the next page

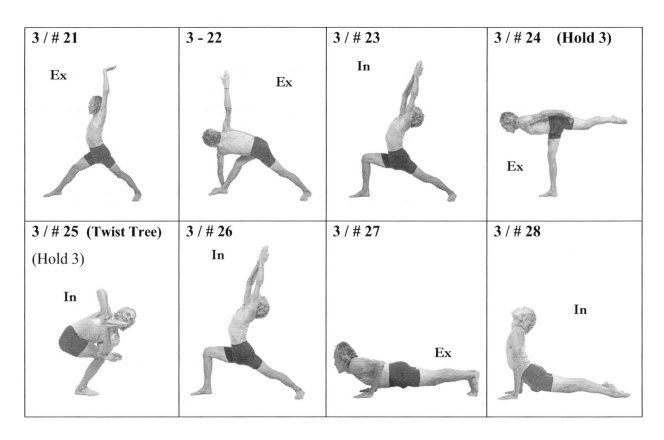

3 / # 21

Ex

3 - 22

Ex

3 / # 23

In

3 / # 24   (Hold 3)

Ex

3 / # 25 (Twist Tree)

(Hold 3)

In

3 / # 26

In

3 / # 27

Ex

3 / # 28

In

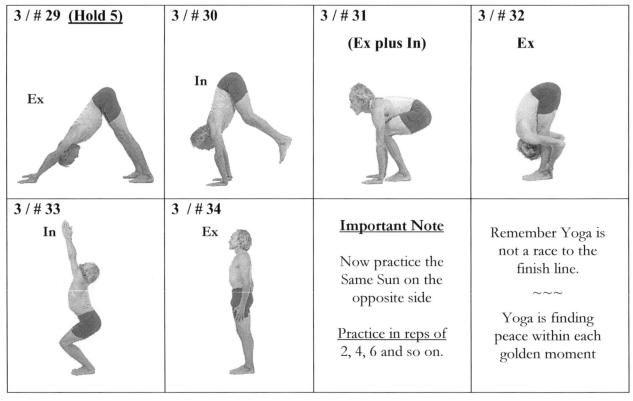

3 / # 29 (Hold 5)

Ex

3 / # 30

In

3 / # 31

(Ex plus In)

3 / # 32

Ex

3 / # 33

In

3 / # 34

Ex

<u>Important Note</u>

Now practice the
Same Sun on the
opposite side

<u>Practice in reps of</u>
2, 4, 6 and so on.

Remember Yoga is
not a race to the
finish line.

~~~

Yoga is finding
peace within each
golden moment

Suggestions for Sun Salutation

At some point in time, you really need to practice your Sun Salutation outdoors, facing the sun, at either sunrise or sunset. This is the way the sacred exercise was designed to be experienced, because it is an honoring, or respect of the sun and truly means much more – the Sun Salutation is to show gratitude for your life on this amazing planet. Energetically speaking, sunrise and sunset are the two most tranquil times of the day, because the energy of the sun - in relationship to where you are located on earth - is either just opening up, or just closing down. These two times of day are the most tranquil, spiritual and inspirational times of day.

~ Sun Salutation - Outdoor Practice ~

When the weather is nice, find a tranquil space in nature and show your gratitude for life
Practicing your Sun Salutation with Mother Nature.

CATEGORY #4 - STANDING POSES   (PG 115- 139)

Cat 4 / # 1 – (*Padangusthasana* and *Padahastasana*):

Padangusthasana: In Sanskrit language *pada* means "foot" while *angustha* means "big toe."
Padahastasana: In Sanskrit language *pada* means for foot while *hasta* means "hand." These two postures are similar, standing forward bend, with a choice of grabbing the big toes, or placing hands under feet.

Benefits:

Helps strengthen abdominal organs, eliminates possibilities of abdominal bloating, constipation, indigestion and other gastric problems. Also stretches the whole backside of the body from the back of the leg muscles to the back of the neck. Variation B gives a nice counter stretch to the wrist, which is well needed in preventing cumulative wrist injuries.

Modifications: Keep the knees bent or place your hands on yoga blocks.

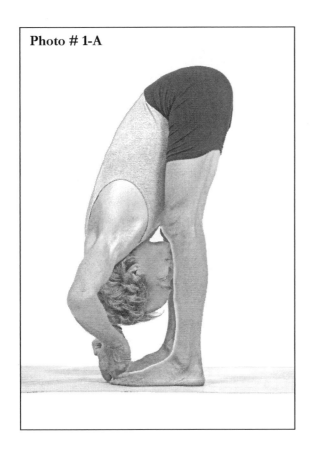

Photo # 1-A

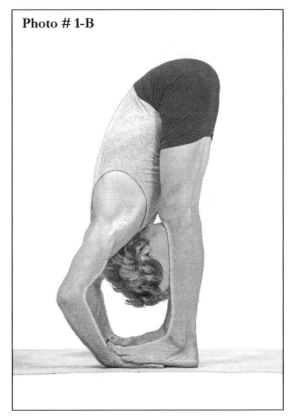

Photo # 1-B

Cautions:

- Back problems: Muscles and Disc

- Neck tension

- Glaucoma

Modifications:

Keep the knees bent or place your hands on yoga blocks.

Vinyasa:

(**Vin # 12** Short Jump Vinyasa) (**Pg 66 – 67**).

Modify – Step instead of jump

Your Body Type - can play a large role in practicing a particular yoga asana.

If you cannot reach your toes – try keeping your knees slightly bent, and place your hands on your thighs, or on a pair of blocks.

Make any modifications to keep your practice safe and progressive.

Instructions: <u>Padangusthasana & Padahastasana - Cat 4 / # 1-A, # 1-B (Pg 115 – 117)</u>.

1. Stand with feet about one foot apart, inhale lifting arms up over your head, then exhale bend forward to grasp big toes with your first two fingers, now inhale looking upward and straighten arms, expanding chest, now exhale and fold forward **(photo 1-A)**.

2. If you are less flexible, bend your knees and grab ankles, or legs, or use a strap. Hold for 5 slow deep breaths.

3. *Padahastasana* This is the sister asana – follow the same instructions, only now you strive to place your hands under your feet **(photo 1-B)**. If less flexible, you may modify by repeating the first variation.

4. To exit… inhale, then release your toes, bend your knees and lift your arms up over your head and return back to standing.

<u>Cat 4 / # 2 - Extended Triangle Pose (*Utthita Trikonasana*):</u>

The word *utthita* means "extended" and *trikona* means "triangle." In this posture you will form an extended triangle with your body.

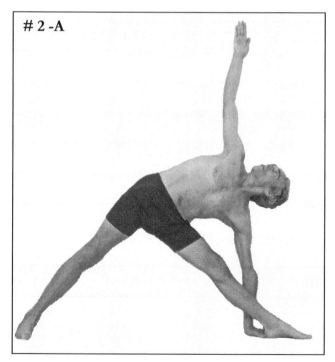

2 -A

Benefits:

This posture strengthens the muscles of your legs, and creates more mobility in your hips. Also serves to stretch the sides of your torso, while teaching balance and coordination.

Cautions:

- Lower back
- Neck tension
- Glaucoma
- Knee injury

Modifications:

Use a block under your supporting hand or rest elbow on knee and keep front knee slightly bent.

Vinyasa:

Take # 13 Wide Jump - **Pg 67**

Then # 14 Triangle Vinyasa- **Pg 68-69**

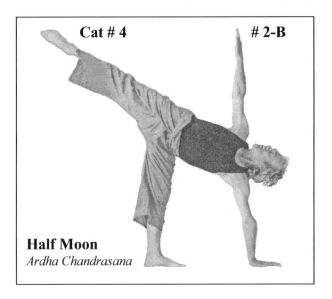

Cat # 4   # 2-B

Half Moon
Ardha Chandrasana

Modifications:

Rest your back on the wall, with block under your supporting hand and front knee slightly bent.

Instructions: Triangle Pose - Cat 4 / # 2 (Pg 117 – 119)

1. Start from a wide standing position, with your feet a little more than shoulders width apart and your arms by your sides.

2. With your body weight evenly distributed between both feet, pivot your left foot outward toward your left side.

3. On an inhalation stretch your left arm outward to your left side, leaning to the left with your torso. Pivot your right foot slightly inward.

4. Try to keep your hips and shoulders open, on the same line as your torso. Continue your exhalation as you tilt your whole torso to your left side lowering your left hand down grabbing the big toe of your left foot. <u>Beg. Use block / Adv. place your hand on the floor.</u>

5. Place your right arm straight up into the air perpendicular to the floor, with your palm facing outward, making a (90-degree angle from your torso with arm) as you gaze upward. Your left fingers grasp onto the big toe of your left foot, or place your hand onto a yoga block, if you are more flexible place your hand on the floor **(photo 2-A).**

6. Hold this position for five complete breaths. Keep your torso extended out over your left leg. Try to keep the chest expanded and your back flat. Turn your vision up toward your left hand, as you gaze up toward the ceiling and lengthen your neck.

7. **Half Moon Pose** – Place your left hand of the floor in front of your left foot, lean forward lifting your right leg up parallel to the floor, or higher, then balance for 5 breaths **(Cat 4, photo # 2-B)**.

8. Repeat the same exercise on the opposite side, and then return to Mountain Posture.

Cat 4 / # 3 - Revolved Triangle Pose (*Parivrtta Trikonasana*):

Parivrtta means "twisted" or "revolved" and *trikona* is a "triangle." In this posture, you will twist your torso around as you form an extended triangle.

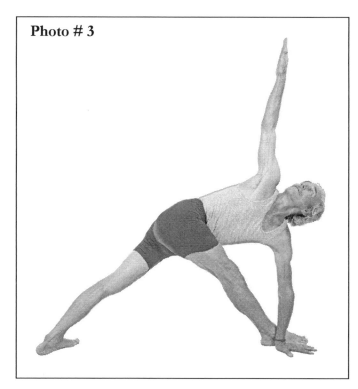

Photo # 3

Benefits:

The Twisted Extended Triangle helps to relieve backaches, tones your spine and strengthens your back and helps to strengthen hamstring, thigh and calf muscles.

Cautions:

- Neck tension
- Glaucoma
- Knee injury
- Ankle stress

Modifications:

Bend your right knee slightly and rest your left elbow onto your right thigh, or place your left hand onto a yoga block - placed next to your right ankle, on the inside or outside of the foot.

Vinyasa: Revolved Triangle - Vin #15 **(Pg 70)**

Instructions: <u>Revolved Triangle Pose - Cat 4 / # 3 (Pg 119 – 120)</u>

1. Start from a wide standing position, with your feet a little more than shoulders' width apart and your arms by your sides.

2. With your body weight evenly distributed between both feet, pivot your right foot outward toward your right side as you lower your left hand to the outside of your right foot, lifting your right hand upward toward the ceiling, drawing one line from your supporting left hand through your shoulders and out your right fingertips **(photo # 3).**

3. Hold this position for five slow deep breaths. Try to keep your hips squared and your torso extended out over your right supporting leg. Move your right hip back and your left shoulder under, lengthen through your neck and keep your vision upward. Hold this position for five complete breaths.

4. When finished, inhale and gracefully circle your extended arms, like a windmill as you return back to standing, then exhale moving on to the opposite side. When finished, inhale and return back to standing, with your arms by your sides, and then relax back to Mountain Posture **(Pg 136 / # 14),** or take a vinyasa onward.

Cat 4 / # 4 - Extended Side Angle Pose (*Utthita Parsvakonasana*):

Utthita means "stretched" or "extended," *parsva* means "side" or "flank" and *kona* relates to an "angle." In this pose you will form an extended side angle with your body.

Benefits:

In the Extended Side Angle Pose, you will strengthen legs, tone ankles, knees, and thighs. This posture can also help to develop your chest and reduce fat around your waist and abdominal area. This pose teaches a combination of strength and softness, grace and power.

Modifications:
Try to place your left elbow onto your left thigh, or use a block under your left hand.

Cautions:

- Ankle stress, Neck tension, or Knee injury.

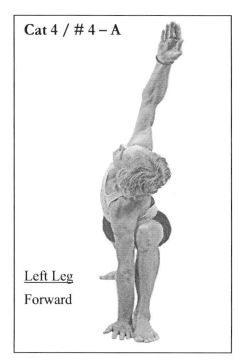

Cat 4 / # 4 – A

Left Leg
Forward

Vinyasa:

Side Angle, Part 1- Vin # 10 – **(Pg 63).**

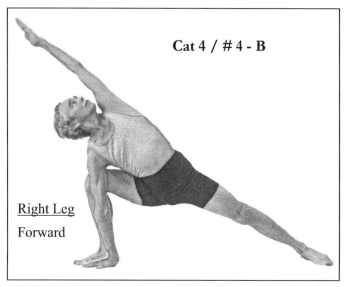

Cat 4 / # 4 - B

Right Leg
Forward

Instructions: Side Angle Pose - Cat 4 / # 4-A, B (Pg 120 – 121)

1. **Left Side # 4-A**: Start from a wide standing position, then on an exhalation start to lunge down onto your left leg, forming a ninety-degree angle with your left knee.

2. Moving deeper, place your left hand on a block, or to the inside of your left foot, with your hand resting onto the floor, as you extend your right arm above your head forming a 45 degree angle, on the same plane as your torso **(photo # 4-A).**

3. From your right extended foot through your torso and out to your left finger-tips you will form a nice 45 degree angle **(photo # 4-A).**

4. Turn your head upward looking up toward the ceiling, trying to look up under your right arm and hold this position for five slow deep breaths.

5. When finished, inhale and stand back up, then repeat the exercise on the right **(# 4-B).**

Cat 4 / # 5 - Twisted Extended Side Angle Pose

(*Parvritta Utthita Parsvakonasana*)

Parvritta means "twisted," or "turned around," and *utthita* means "stretched" or "extended."
Parsva means "side" or "flank," and *kona* means "angle." In this pose you will form a twisted, extended side angle with your body.

Benefits:

In the Extended Side Angle Pose you will strengthen legs, tone ankles, knees, and thighs. Your spine will be toned and invigorated. This posture can also help to develop your chest and reduce fat around your waist and abdominal area.

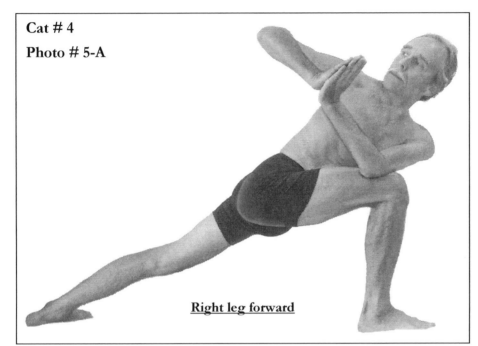

Cat # 4

Photo # 5-A

Right leg forward

Cautions:

- Tight Calves
- Ankle injury
- Neck tension
- Knee injury

Twisted Side Angle-
Vinyasa -
Part 2 -Vin # 11
(Pg 64-66)

Modifications:

Try to place your left knee on the ground, resting onto a folded blanket and keep the upper body twisted.

Less Intense: Stay with the hands in prayer option, and skip the Bound Option # 5-B.

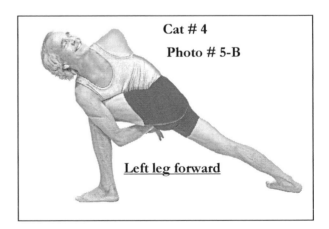

Cat # 4

Photo # 5-B

Left leg forward

Instructions: <u>Twisted Side Angle Pose - Cat 4 / # 5-A, B (Pg 121 – 123)</u>

1. From a standing position with feet more than shoulders width apart, pivot your right foot outward about ninety degrees and your left foot inward about thirty degrees.

2. Now lunge down onto you right leg as you twist your upper body to the right and try to rest your left elbow on your right thigh with hands in prayer fashion. <u>Beginners: use a wall for support, or rest your left knee onto the floor.</u>

3. Try to form one line of energy from your left extended leg through your torso and out the top of your head. Move your right hip back and your left shoulder under **(photo # 5-A)**. Hold this for 5 complete breaths, then come to standing and repeat on left side.

4. **Advanced:** reach your right arm under your left bent knee and try grasping your left wrist behind your back in the *bound* Twisted Side Angle **(photo 5-B)** Demo pose is on left side.

5. When finished, on an inhalation begin to straighten your left leg, as you return back to standing and then repeat to practice on the right side.

Cat 4 / # 6 - Expanded Foot Pose (*Prasarita Padottanasana*):

Pada means "foot" and *prasarita* means "spread, expanded," or "extended," In this posture you will be stretching and moving energy in several different directions at once.

Benefits:

This posture creates strength and flexibility in your hamstrings, calves, and ankles while bringing an easy blood supply to your torso and brain. The pose allows for more range of motion in your shoulders and also assists in creating an alternative for those who have not yet accomplished the Headstand.

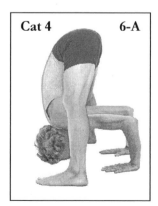
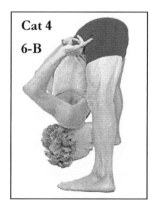
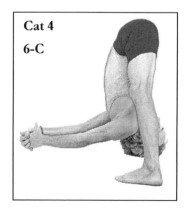

Modifications: If the hands do not reach the floor, either walk the feet wider apart or place yoga block under the hands, or head, with knees bent slightly.

Vinyasa: <u>Chi Flow Vinyasa (Vin # 9), **(Pg 62 - 63)** (Use In and out of asana)</u>

Instructions: <u>Expanded Foot Pose - Cat 4 / # 6 (Pg 123 – 125)</u>

1. Stand with your spine straight and shoulders back, your feet slightly more than shoulders width apart. Turn your toes slightly inward and heels outward, grounding yourself into the Earth with the outsides of your feet.

2. Now start your exhalation, lowering your hands down between your feet and trying to place your head down between your hands **(photo #6-A).** Beg. Modification **(Pg 123).**

3. Place your wrist up under your elbows and make your arms parallel with one another. If you are more flexible, you can move your head back beyond the centerline of your torso.

4. Hold this position for five deep breaths. When you are finished, inhale bending knees and return to standing. Then proceed with the next 3 variations.

5. **Option # 6-B:** Practice the same exercise with hands on your hips **(photo #6-B).**

6. **Option # 6-C:** Interlace your fingers, with arms extended behind your back, exhale as you hinge forward at your waist lowering your head to the floor and your arms behind your back, opening your chest and shoulders. Hold this position for five complete breaths **(Photo #6-C).** Modify – **Hold a strap between your hands**

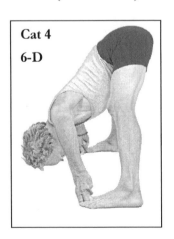

Cat 4
6-D

7. **<u>Option # 6-D:</u>** Exhale hinging forward and grab the big toes of your extended feet with your first two fingers. Hold this for 5 complete breaths **(photo #6-D).** To Modify - bend knees.

<u>Cat 4 / # 7 - Pyramid Pose (*Parsvottanasana*):</u>

Parsvottanasana means "intense side stretch." in this yoga posture you will be practicing a combination of triangle and standing forward bend, as you form a pyramid shape.

Modifications: (Pyramid Pose)

If you cannot reach your chest to thigh, bend your right knee slightly and move out over the thigh. If you cannot place hands in prayer or hold wrist – just grab elbows behind your back.

Cautions: Knee, Hip and Shoulder injury.

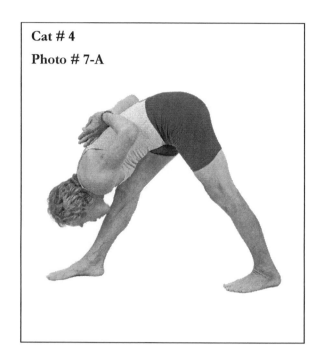

Cat # 4

Photo # 7-A

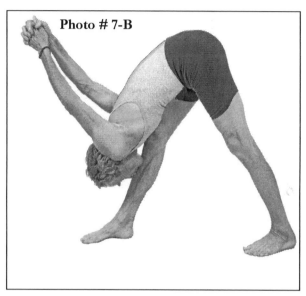

Photo # 7-B

Vinyasa: <u>Short Jump Vinyasa (Vin # 12), or step, or jump, to the side</u> (**Pg 66 - 67**)

Benefits:

Teaches balance, at the same time, promotes flexibility and strength. This posture stretches the back side of your leg muscles, expands the chest, while strengthening your ankles and legs. In addition, your hips and wrists are also given a gentle opening.

Instructions: **Pyramid Pose - Cat 4 / # 7-A, B (Pg 124 – 126)**

1. From a standing position, with feet about 2 feet apart, (pivot your right foot and hips to the right side) and try to square your hips. Keeping the back foot flat on the floor, with the toes facing slightly forward.

2. Bend forward and try to move your chest toward your right thigh, reaching torso out over your extended right knee. Beg. - Leave hands resting on hips.

3. **Beg**: Round your spine moving the chin toward your right knee, and relax.

   Beg: Stay here in this preparatory stage, breathing deeply for 5 breaths.

4. More flexible – try to place your hands in prayer fashion behind your back **(photo # 7-A)**, or for another variation, interlace your fingers and straighten the arms down toward the floor **(photo # 7-B)**.

5. To come out - bend the right knee and exhale, release arms inhale and return to standing. Then practice the same exercise on the opposite side.

Cat 4 / # 8 - Sun Dial Pose (*Utthita Hasta Padangusthasana*):

The word *utthita* means "extended," *hasta* means "hand," and *pandangustha* means "big toe." In this posture you will extend your hand holding onto your big toe. I prefer to call this posture the "Sun Dial" as you take a striking resemblance to this ancient clock.

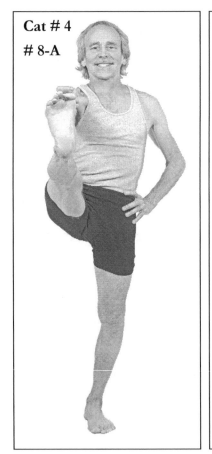

Cat # 4
8-A

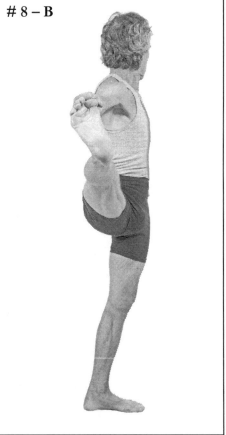

8 – B

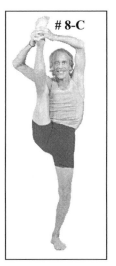

8-C

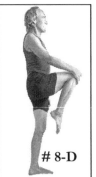

8-D

Benefits:

This pose teaches balance and poise, while strengthening your ankles, and muscles of your legs. Helps relieve stiff hips and firm's abdominal muscles.

Cautions:

- Ankle

- Low back injury

- Knee injury

> **Cross-training** - to gain more balance for Sun Dial Pose try practicing your yoga outdoors, with uneven ground and diverse landscape. You will improve your balance and find peace in nature and warmth in your heart.

Modifications:

Keep your right knee bent, and grab your right knee, as an alternative to grasping toes, or use a strap to extend your reach. Another option is to use the wall for support.

Vinyasa:

Use Sundial Vinyasa

Vinyasa # 8

This is soft / less power

(Pg 61 – 62)

> With the Sundial Vinyasa strive to move precise and yet free flowing, as a moving meditation. Time your motion in sync - with your breathing.

Instructions: Sun Dial Pose - Cat 4 / # 8-A, B, C (Pg 126 – 128)

1. Start from a position standing up straight with feet about (one-half foot apart).

2. Now exhale and place your left hand on your left hip as you bend your right leg, taking hold of your right big toe, or knee with your right hand, and straighten your right leg **(photo # 8-A).   Beg. Option:** Hold Knee **(photo # 8-D, Pg 126).**

3. Strive to keep your back straight and your hips squared, hold this position for five complete breaths.

4. Now exhale and move your right leg to the right side of your body, as you look to the left **(photo # 8-B).** Hold this position for an additional five complete breaths.

5. Then, **(Adv Option),** bring leg back to the front and lift higher **(photo# 8-C),** now lower leg parallel to the floor without hands and hold for another 5 breaths.

6. When finished, exhale and bend your right leg and return to a standing position

7. Repeat the same instructions, this time with your left leg extended.

Cat 4 / # 9 - Half Bound Lotus Standing Forward Bend:

Ardha Baddha Padmottanasan in sanskrit *ardha*, means "half" and *baddha* means "bound" and *padma* means "lotus." Then *ut* means "intense" and *tan* meaning "stretch" with asana meaning "pose." Half Bound Lotus Standing Forward Fold is a deep hip opener and hamstring stretch that can be challenging even for more advanced students. The pose can definitely be intense, especially for the knees, so it is important to be certain that you are not creating injury when you practice this posture.

Benefits:

In this pose, you will stretch and strengthen the hips, hamstrings, shoulders, ankles, and knees. It helps to cleanse the liver and spleen, and improves and regulates the digestive system. This pose also improves circulation to the brain.

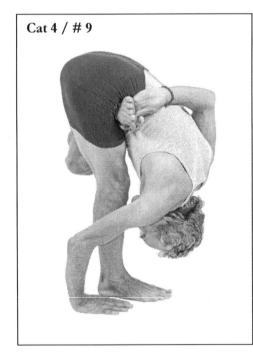

Cat 4 / # 9

Modifications:

A) - Use a block under your right hand.

B) - Use a strap to extend reach for your ½ lotus.

C) - Chose not to bend forward.

D) – Keep right knee bent on supporting leg

Cautions:

• Knee or hip injury

• Headaches, glaucoma

• High or low blood pressure

Vinyasa: More power (Vin # 2-C) **Pg 53** or (Vin # 4) **Pg 55**

Instructions: Half Lotus Standing Forward Bend - Cat 4 / # 9 (Pg 128 – 129)

1. Begin standing up straight in the mountain pose with your arms at your sides.

2. Now you can begin to shift your weight onto your right foot and ground down firmly as you stand on you right foot only.

3. Slowly bend your left knee up toward your hips and with awareness, place you left ankle on your right thigh, or in (1/2 lotus). You can modify, by just simply bending your knee.

4. **Advanced**: Hold onto your left foot with your left hand behind your back in Half Bound Lotus**.**

5. Inhale and lift your right arm straight up, then exhale as you fold forward, hinging at the hips, and placing your right hand on the ground. Draw your chin toward your chest and concentrate on bringing your forehead to your shin bone **(photo # 9)**.

6. Hold for five breaths, then on an inhalation, bend your right knee and lift your torso back to an upright position. Release your lotus foot slowly and with awareness returning back to the floor and to Mountain Pose. Now repeat on the same sequence on the opposite side.

Cat 4 / # 10 - Warrior Pose (*Virabhadrasana*):

The word, *Virabhadra* means "hero" or "warrior" and gets its name from the powerful, presence you embrace when practicing these strong asanas. In Hindu legend, this posture is dedicated to *Virabhadra*, the powerful warrior hero who was created by *Siva* by extracting him from his matted hair.

Benefits:

All variations tone and strengthen leg muscles, expand your chest, and help you develop deep, powerful breathing, and good balance. Also relieves tension in your shoulders and back as well as strengthens your ankles. Warrior 3 adds an extra balance factor.

Cautions:

- Weak or injured Knee / Tight Ankles

Modifications:

(Warrior 1 and 2) – Do not lunge so deeply, and, or, leave your hands on your hips.

(Warrior 3) – Rest your extended hands on the wall to assist with balance and keep the knee on your supporting leg slightly bent.

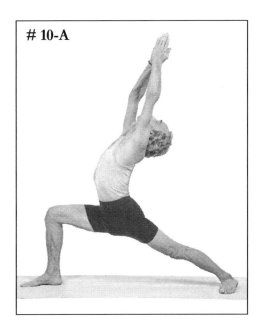

10-A

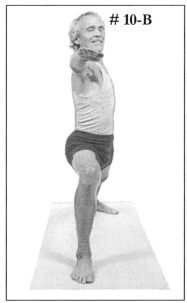

10-B

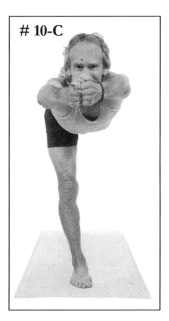

10-C

Vinyasa:

(Choose one method)

A) – Use any Sun Salutation flow **(Pg 104 – 111)** to enter and exit this Warrior Pose.

B) – Or - Simply step forward from Downward Facing Dog **(Pg 191)** to enter the pose.

C) – Or - From Mountain Pose take one big step forward and lunge deep to Warrior Pose.

Instructions:

Warrior 1 Pose - Cat 4 / # 10-A (Pg 130 - 131) -

1. From a wide standing position, lunge down on your right leg with your knee over your heel and thigh parallel to the floor.

2. Square your hips and shoulders forward toward your right foot, your arms are extended straight up over your head, with palms together and your gaze up toward your thumbs. If

your shoulders and neck are very tight, leave your hands about one foot apart and gaze forward, but strive to look upward with hands together **(photo # 10-A)**.

3. Hold this position for five complete breaths. When finished, hold your deep, powerful leg stance, and then move on to the instructions for Warrior II listed below.

(Warrior 2) - Cat 4 / # 10-B (Pg 130 - 131)

1. From Warrior I, open your hips, shoulders and torso -right hip forward, and left hip back. At the same time lower your arms down to rest parallel to the floor, on the same line as your torso, with palms facing downward.

2. Your right knee is still bent at 90 degrees with your knee over your heel. Lengthen through your finger-tips in opposite directions. Your gaze should be forward, parallel to the floor out over your right fingers. Stand very strong and yet relaxed, holding this posture for an additional five complete breaths **(photo # 10-B)**.

3. When finished… inhale, straighten your legs, and lift your torso back to the center, then exhale and flow down to Warrior I and II on the opposite side. Follow the same instructions only this time lunging with your left leg. When finished, move on to the instructions for Warrior 3, or relax into Mountain Pose.

(Warrior 3) - Cat 4 / # 10-C (Pg 130 - 131)

1. Warrior 3 is based within the same strong grounded standing posture as in Warrior 1 and 2, only this time you will balance on one leg. This posture was named for the three avenues of energy flow: your arms point forward, one leg backward, and one leg as a supporting foot.

2. Start this posture from Warrior 1 **(photo # 10-A)**. Now lean forward and try to balance on your right foot, as you extend arms and torso forward and left leg backward, as you keep them parallel to the floor **(photo #10-C)**.

3. Hold this position for five, slow deep breaths. When finished, on an exhalation, bend your right knee and slowly lower your left foot back to the floor, returning to the Mountain posture and relax.

4. Repeat the same exercise, only this time balance on your left leg and extend your right leg behind you.

Cat 4 / #11 - Chair Pose (*Utkatasana*):

Utkatasana means "powerful" or "fierce" and in this asana you will embrace power and resemble the image of a chair.

Benefits:

Chair pose greatly strengthens the lower body while stretching the upper back and shoulders, while invigorating and energizing the whole body with power. If you practice Twisted Chair variation you also receive a great spinal toner.

Modifications:

If the feet are hips width apart you can place a yoga block between the thighs to help keep the knees pointing forward. Some will find it beneficial to elevate the heels with a rolled up towel or yoga wedge.

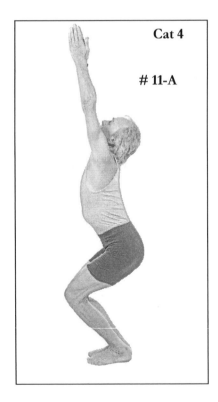

Cat 4

11-A

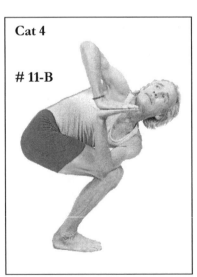

Cat 4

11-B

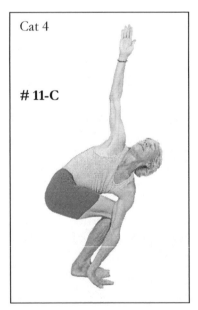

Cat 4

11-C

Cautions:

Weakness or injury to the Hips, Knees, Back or Shoulders.

Vinyasa:

Depending on where you came from and where you are going. Move mindfully on an inhalation from Mountain Pose **(Pg 136),** or enter and exit through a full Sun Salutation **(Pg 104 – 111).**

Instructions: Chair Pose – Cat 4 / # 11 (Pg 132 – 133)

1. Start in Mountain Pose **(Pg 136, # 14)** with the feet either together, or hips distance apart. Now bend the knees, squatting down. Reach the hips down and back as if you were going to sit on the edge of a chair, at the same time lifting the arms up over your head.

2. The gaze can be upward beyond the hands, or parallel to the floor. Avoid bringing the hips lower than the level of the knees and make sure that the knees are pointing straight ahead.

3. Hold this pose for 5 breaths **(photo # 11-A).** When finished exhale and slowly stand back up, or move into a vinyasa to the next asana.

4. **(Variation) Twisted Chair:** If you choose to practice the Twisted Chair Pose, twist your upper body to the right, placing hands in prayer with left elbow, outside of right knee, in **(# 11-B)** or lower one arm down and the other arm upward **(photo # 11-C).**

Cat 4 / # 12 - Dancer Pose (*Natarajasana*):

Natarajasana means "king dancer" and in this pose you will demonstrate the poise, flexibility and grace of a dancer.

Benefits:

This asana opens the shoulders, chest, and hips, as it stretches and strengthens the thighs, ankles, and abdomen. Also inspires greater flexibility in your spine, shoulders, and hamstrings. The Dancer pose also stretches the entire front of the body, while strengthening the back muscles, which improves posture.

Cat # 4 / Photo # 12 -A

Balance on Right Leg

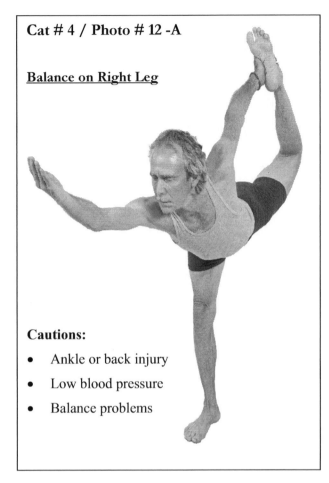

Cautions:

- Ankle or back injury
- Low blood pressure
- Balance problems

Vinyasa: Inhale to lengthen, in Mountain Pose -Then exhale into the Dancer pose.

Modifications:
Place your right arm on the wall for support and balance. Use a strap around back ankle to extend reach.

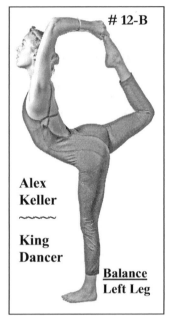

12-B

Alex
Keller
~~~~~
King
Dancer

**Balance
Left Leg**

Instructions: <u>Dancer Pose - Cat 4 / # 12-A, B (Pg 133 - 134)</u>

1. Start in Mountain Pose **(Pg 136, # 14)** with your feet together and your arms at your sides then shift your weight onto your right foot.

2. Bend your left knee and bring your left heel toward your left buttock. Reach your left hand down and clasp your left foot's inner ankle, as right arm extends forward.

3. Lean forward, extending your left leg backward and upward **(photo # 12-A).**

4. Hold for five breaths, then slowly return to Mountain Pose **(Pg 136)**. Then repeat the pose on the opposite side.

5. **<u>Advanced Option (King Dancer):</u>** Hold your foot with both hands, extending your foot upward toward the back of your head **(photo # 12-B).** Demo pose is left leg balance.

Cat 4 / # 13 - Eagle Pose (*Garudasana*):

Garudasana means "eagle," but can also mean "devourer," relating to being able to fight off negative energy. This asana is a standing balance pose that requires and develops focus, strength, and serenity. When you accomplish this asana you will resemble the energy of a confident eagle.

Benefits:

Eagle Pose stretches the shoulders and upper back while strengthening the thighs, hips, ankles, and calves. It builds balance, calm focus, and concentration. The dynamic balancing aspect of the pose can help to protect your knees against future injury.

Modifications:

If you can't yet weave your arms and legs together, just take it easy and do the best you can and try resting the big toe of your raised foot on a yoga block. Beginners and those having trouble balancing can practice this pose against a wall.

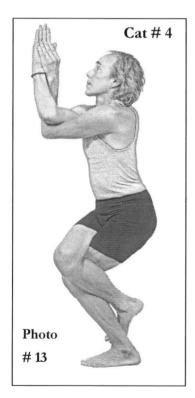

Cat # 4

Photo # 13

Cautions:

- Knee injury
- Pregnancy
- Poor Balance
- Tight Ankles

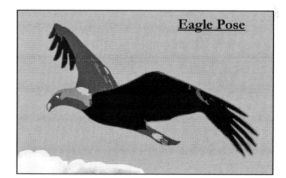

Eagle Pose

Vinyasa: Start in Mountain Pose (Pg 136), move arms and legs, slowly and mindfully, in unison on an inhalation and then exhale as you arrive in the asana.

Instructions: Eagle Pose - Cat 4 / # 13 (Pg 135 - 136):

1. Begin standing in Mountain Pose **(Pg 136)** with your arms at your sides.

2. Bend your knees and balance on your left foot, then place your right thigh over your left thigh, right arm over left. Fix your gaze at a point in front of you. Hook the top of your right foot behind your right calf muscle, or place your foot on a yoga block.

3. Extend your arms in front of your body, resting your right elbow onto of your left bicep, gazing at the tips of your thumbs for 5 breaths **(photo # 13, Pg 135).**

Cat 4 / # 14 - Mountain Pose (*Tadasana*):

The Sanskrit word *Tadasana* refers to a "mountain" and in this *asana* you will stand tall and yet grounded like a mountain.

Benefits:

Teaches balance and self-confidence, improves posture and, when practiced regularly, can help reduce back pain. Tadasana can also strengthen leg muscles and buttocks.

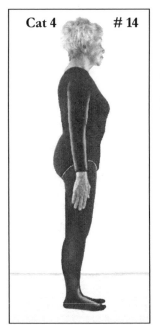

Cat 4   # 14

Modifications:

If you have trouble balancing, stand with your feet six inches apart (or wider) and you can also stand against the wall. Women who are pregnant should widen their stances as much as necessary to feel stable.

Cautions:

- Poor balance
- Dizziness

* Pose Model: (Violet Swenson / Mother)

Instructions: Mountain Pose - Cat 4 / # 14 (Pg 136 - 137)

1. Stand with your feet together and your arms at your sides. Press your weight evenly across the balls and arches of your feet.

2. Draw down through your heels and straighten your legs. Ground your feet firmly into the earth, pressing evenly across all four corners of both feet.

3. Tuck in your tailbone slightly, but don't round your lower back, bringing your pelvis to its neutral position

4. Keep shoulder blades back and yet relaxed as you elongate your neck. Softly gaze forward toward the horizon line. Hold this pose for 5 breaths **(photo # 14).**

Vinyasa: Start in Mountain Pose, close your eyes and visualize the pose, enter without vinyasa, or use – Hard Vin: # 2-A, B, and C **(Pg 53-54)** / Soft Vin: # 4 **(Pg 55 – 57).**

Cat 4 / # 15 - Horse Pose (*Vatyanasana*):

Vatyan means "horse" and in this *asana* you will somewhat resemble the posture and energy of a horse, -feel the power and freedom of wild horses roaming free.

Benefits:

Promotes flexibility in the hips and ankles as you strengthen leg muscles and promotes good balance.

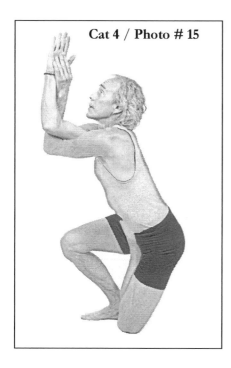

Cat 4 / Photo # 15

Cautions

- Knee injury,
- Ankle Injury

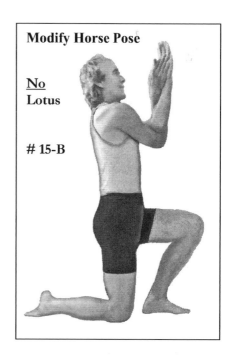

Modify Horse Pose

<u>No</u> **Lotus**

15-B

Modifications:

Do not place left foot in ½ lotus; instead just rest your knee on the floor, placed behind your heel. For sensitive or injured knees, place a pad under your right knee **(Pg 137, photo # 15-B).**

Vinyasa:

From Mountain Pose **(Pg 136, photo #14)** all in one smooth motion, (inhale follow Part 1 and exhale follow Part 2) of the instructions. To exit, inhale as to lift your arms as a bird's wings, stand back up and return to Mountain Pose then exhale.

Instructions: Horse Pose - Cat 4 / # 15 (Pg 137 - 138)

1. Start in Mountain Pose **(Pg 136, photo # 14),** balance on your right foot as you bend your left knee, and step back with your left foot about 2 feet and allowing your left knee to rest on the floor near your right ankle. **Beginners use this leg position.**

2. Lift your arms in front of the torso, bending elbows and allow your right elbow to rest on top of your left bicep, as you wrap one arm around the other. **Beg. & Inter:** stay in this position for 5 breaths on each side.

3. **Advanced** – Practice this asana with left leg in ½ lotus position and left knee resting on the floor, next to your right ankle **(photo # 15).** Hold 5 breaths and then exit slowly and mindfully back to Mountain Pose. **Option** - Place pillow under left knee.

Cat 4 / # 16 - Tree Pose (*Vrksasana*):

In Sanskrit, the word *vrksa*, means "tree" and the word *asana* means "pose." In this simple and fun asana you will take on the essence and energy of a tree as you plant your yoga roots into the energy of earth. Tree Pose, with its calming and meditative benefits, is like a standing variation of a seated meditation posture.

Modifications:

If you are unable to bring your foot to rest on your thigh, then you can rest your foot alongside your calf muscle or place a yoga block under your right foot. If you are very unsteady, try practicing this asana with your back against a wall, or one hand on the wall for extra support.

Option:

For a greater challenge, once you are in the asana, balance on one foot with hands over your heart, or overhead – then try to close your eyes and find your internal balance.

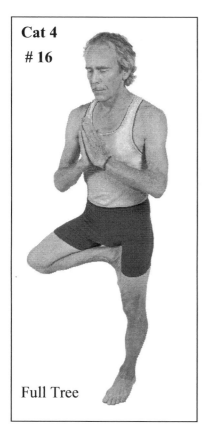

Cat 4
16

Full Tree

Cautions:

- Headaches
- Insomnia
- Blood pressure
- Dizzy

In Photo # 16-A – Try

The Small Tree: Balance-
on your toes of right foot, with left leg bent, ankle resting on the right thigh / hands in prayer on head.

Vinyasa: Inhale lifting your right foot and both arms, then exhale moving into the pose.
Or Vin # 1 **(Pg 53-54 /** Vin # 4 **(Pg 55 – 57)**

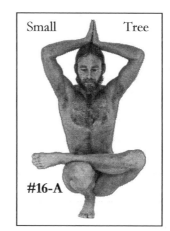

Small   Tree

#16-A

Instructions: Tree Pose - Cat 4 / # 16 (Pg 138 - 139)

1. Start from standing in Mountain Pose with your arms at your sides. Distribute your weight evenly across both feet, grounding down equally through both feet.
2. Now move your weight to your left foot, as you bend your right knee, and place your right foot to rest upon your left inner thigh, or on alongside the inner left knee.
3. Rest your hands in prayer fashion over your heart or with palms together up over your head.
4. Fix your gaze softly on one, unmoving point in front of you.
5. Push down through your left foot, as your right foot rests gently on your left inner thigh **(photo # 16)**. Try to keep Hips open.
6. Hold for 5 breaths and then relax back to Mountain Pose, and repeat on the opposite side. When finished, move through a vinyasa, or return to Mountain Pose and relax.

CATEGORY # 5 - INVERTED POSTURES (PG 140 – 147)

(Headstand, Shoulder Stand and Counter Stretches)

Cat 5 / #1 - Headstand (*Sirsasana*):

The Sanskrit word *Sirsa* means "head." In this posture you will balance on your head, supported by your arms. The Headstand is considered to be one of the main postures, due to its wonderful calming and relaxing effect on your whole body. The Headstand is an intermediate to advance posture, however anyone can practice the preliminary variations.

Benefits:

The Headstand posture helps you develop balance, self-confidence, and forearm strength. Moderate inverted poses assist to bring oxygenated blood to the heart and brain. Combined with yoga deep breathing,- which increases the oxygen supply to your blood,- inverted poses will leave you feeling refreshed and at peace.

Modifications: Keep one or both feet on the ground **(photo #1-B),** or use a wall for support.

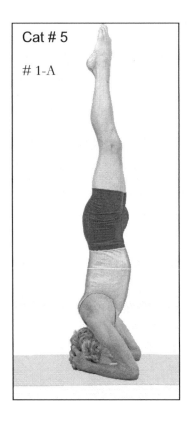

Cat # 5

1-A

Cautions:

Injury to Eye, or Neck, Menstrual cycle and high Blood Pressure.

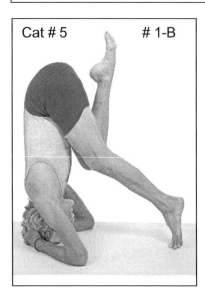

Cat # 5   # 1-B

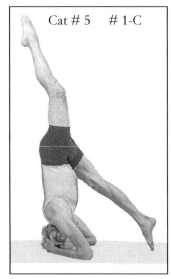

Cat # 5   # 1-C

Headstand Variations:

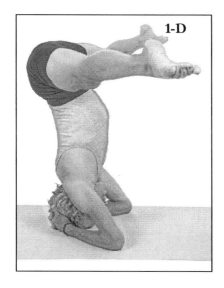
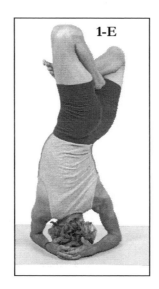
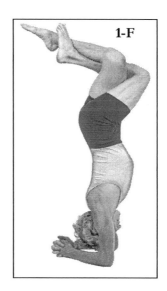

Vinyasa:

(Vin # 4) – Missing Link up **(Pg 55 – 57)** following instructions 1- 3, then take the Headstand foundation (Instruction # 3 below).

Instructions: Headstand - Cat 5 / # 1 (Pg 140 - 142)

1. Start your Headstand from a Thunderbolt Pose **(Pg 92, photo # 6),** resting on knees.

2. Now, resting on hands and knees, lean forward while lifting hips up off your calves; then, supported with hands in front of knees, form a table top, resting on hands and knees. Torso, arms and legs form 90 degree angles.

3. Then place your elbows, on the floor in front of your knees, interlacing your fingers, but leaving your hands cupped, to allow your head to rest in your palms.

4. Support most of your weight on your elbows, making sure to keep your elbows close to your head as you straighten your legs slowly, placing more weight on your head.

5. Slowly walk your feet up toward your face, without pushing yourself over backward, until your torso is almost vertical to the floor.

6. Now bend your right knee and try to lift your right foot up off the floor **(photo # 1-B).**

7. If you are confident about your balance, try the next step into headstand with your back against a wall for added support.

8. Lift one foot at a time and continue into full headstand pose **(photo # 1-A)**. Hold this position five to twenty breaths.

9. **Option (1-C)** - Split Straight Legs, leaving One Foot on the Floor **(photo # 1-C)**.

10. **Option (1-D)** – Split Legs, Right to Left **(photo # 1-D)**.

11. **Option (1-E)** – Headstand Lotus, Arch and Twist **(photo # 1-E)**

12. **Option (1-F)** – Flying Eagle Headstand **(photo # 1-F)**.

13. When finished come down slowly, on an exhalation by bending your knees into your chest and lowering your torso back down onto your thighs into Child's Pose and relax for a few slow deep breaths.

Cat 5 / # 2 - Shoulder Stand (*Salamba Sarvangasana*):

Salamba means "propped" or "supported," *sarva* means "whole" or "complete" and *anga* means "limb" or "body." In this posture, you will support your body with your hands and elbows. This pose has acquired the appropriate name of Shoulder Stand, as you will balance your body on your shoulders.

Benefits:

The Shoulder Stand stimulates the endocrine system and the thyroid and parathyroid glands are given a tune up. Due to being upside down you will receive an easy blood supply to your heart and brain, and help to reverse the effects of varicose veins. When you come out of Shoulder Stand, you will feel refreshed and rejuvenated.

Modifications:

If you have a sensitive neck, place a blanket under your shoulders to create a few inches of additional elevation. If you find it difficult to support yourself in a Shoulder Stand, start your shoulder stand with your feet on a wall. In this manner you can bend your knees and push against the wall with your feet to give yourself added support.

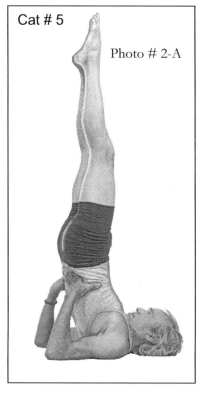

Cat # 5

Photo # 2-A

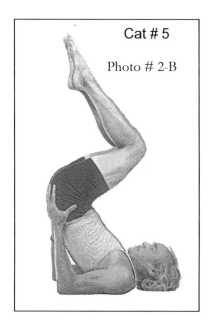

Cat # 5

Photo # 2-B

Cautions:

- Injured neck
- Glaucoma
- Eye injury
- Moon Cycle

Options

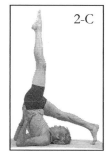

2-C

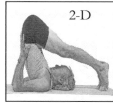

2-D

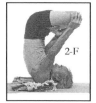

2-E

2-F

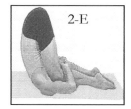

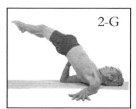

2-G

Vinyasa: Lying on your back – inhale, stretching your arms and legs long, (as if you just woke up), then exhale and move into the Shoulder Stand Pose.

Instructions: <u>**Shoulder Stand - Cat 5 / # 2 (Pg 142 - 144)**</u>

1. Start in Corpse Pose **(Pg # 206, Cat 10 - Photo # 1).** On an exhalation, bend your knees while pulling them into your chest. Then place your hands on the floor palms facing downward on the outside of your hips.

2. Now lift your hips as you bend your elbows and place hands on your hips or buttocks, as you lift your torso upward **(photo # 2-B)**. Beginners stay in this position and hold for 5 – 15 breaths.

3. Place your elbows behind your back so that they are parallel to one another, tucking your chin down into your chest

4. **Intermediate students** - try to lift your torso up higher and form a more vertical line with your torso and legs, placing hands on your back **(photo # 2-A)**. If you have any tension in the neck, elevate your shoulders on a folded blanket. Hold for 5 – 15 breaths.

5. **Option (2-C) One Leg Plough:** Lower right leg to the floor, as you keep both legs straight **(photo # 2-C)**. Hold for 5 – 10 breaths and repeat with left leg.

6. **Option (2-D) Plough Pose (Halasana):** Lower both legs to the floor, as you try to keep both legs straight **(photo # 2-D)**. Hold for 5 - 10 breaths.

7. **Option (2-E) Knees by Ears (Karnipidasana):** Lower both knees to the floor, resting to the outside of your ears **(photo # 2-E)**. Hold for 5 breaths.

8. **Option (2-F) Lotus Shoulder Stand (Padma Sarvangasana):** Place your feet in lotus or modified lotus position, with hands on back or supporting under knees. Many will find this pose more comfortable, and help avoid injury by elevating the shoulders with a folded blanket **(photo # 2-F)**. Hold for 5 breaths.

9. **Option (2-G) Shoulder Stand Arch:** Place your left hand and arm on floor to your left side, then arch your body to the right **(photo # 2-F)**. Hold 5 breaths. Repeat on left side.

    When finished - relax into corpse position for few breaths and prepare for Fish Posture.

Cat 5 / # 3 Bridge Pose (*Setu Bandasana*):

In Sanskrit *Setu* means a "dam" or "bridge," *Bandha* means "lock" and *Asana* is "pose."
In this pose you will resemble a bridge over a river

Benefits:

Bridge Pose stretches the chest, neck, and spine as it calms the brain and helps alleviate stress and mild depression. This asana also stimulates abdominal organs, lungs, and improves digestion. In addition, Bridge Pose helps relieve the symptoms of menopause. This asana relieves menstrual discomfort when practiced with support & Reduces fatigue, and insomnia.

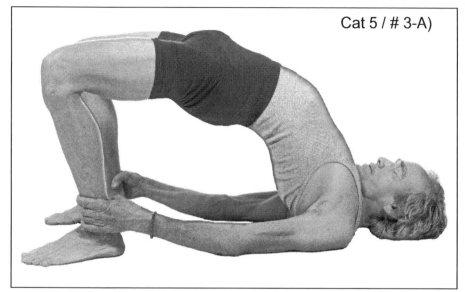

Cat 5 / # 3-A)

Cautions:

- Neck injury
- Shoulder injury

Vinyasa: (Hard)
From Shoulder
Stand - float down.
(Easy) from Corpse
Pose bend the knees,
then plant feet and
lift your hips.

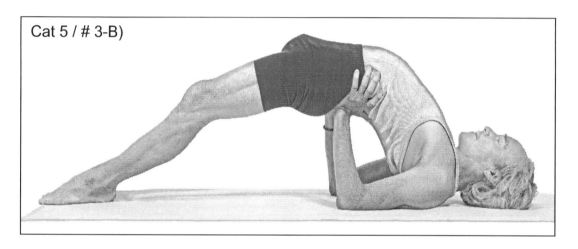

Cat 5 / # 3-B)

Modifications: Leave hands resting on the floor, and try elevating the sacrum with a large bolster or blocks and strive to lift up and off the support.

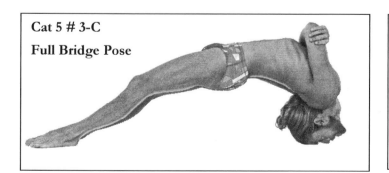

Cat 5 # 3-C

Full Bridge Pose

 # 3-C / Cautions –

This pose can be dangerous to your neck, best for advanced with an experience teacher. Lay down on a bolster with your head off the edge on the floor, to support your total body weight. Use caution, it is not necessary to practice this pose.

Instructions: Bridge Pose – Cat 5 / # 3 (Pg 144 – 146)

1. Start by lying on your back in Corpse Pose **(Pg 206, Cat 10 / # 1).**

2. Bend your knees with feet flat on the floor about hips distance apart, with hands resting by your sides - palms facing downward.

3. Exhale as you lift hips upward, pushing down with feet. Lift your buttocks until the thighs are about parallel to the floor and try to keep your knees directly over the heels.

4. Hands can remain on the floor, or place hands onto your back for support or if you have the flexibility grasp onto ankles with hands **(photo # 3-A).**

5. Hold for 5 – 10 breaths then relax back to corpse pose, or move through a vinyasa.

6. **Option (9-B):** Place your hands up under hips and/or lower back as you extend your feet away from your head with feet flat and legs straight **(photo # 3-B).**

7. **Option (9-C) Full Bridge:** Rest on your head with arms over chest. **(Caution, Advanced)**

Cat 5 / # 4 - Fish Posture (*Matsyasana*):

Matsya means a "fish." This posture is dedicated to the Hindu legend of *Matsya*, the fish incarnation of *Visnu*, who is the "source and maintainer of all things." This posture is also used as a wonderful counter stretch for the headstand.

Benefits:

In the Fish Posture, your thyroid gland is rejuvenated, due to the stretching of your neck. Your chest is expanded and helps greatly if you suffer from shallow breathing. This asana also serves to open the hips and release tension from your shoulders.

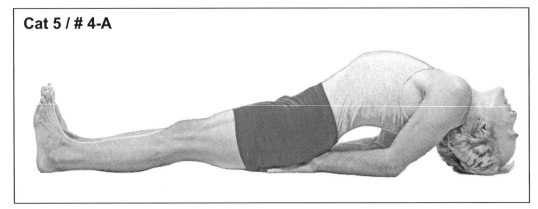

Cat 5 / # 4-A

Cautions:
Neck injury
Eye injury

Instructions: <u>Fish Pose – Cat 5 / # 4 (Pg 146 – 147)</u>

1. Start from the Corpse Posture **(Pg 206),** with your legs extended, as you sit on top of your hands, palms facing downward.

2. Now arch your back up off the floor expanding your chest, as you push down with your elbows, and hands **(photo # 4-A).** Hold this position for five very slow deep breaths.

3. **Option (4-B) Lotus Fish:** Place feet in lotus and rest hands on thighs, or grasp toes.

4. **Option (4-C) Flying Fish:** Lift straight arms and legs on a 30-degree angle.

5. **5.** When you finish exhale and return to the Corpse Position to relax.

Vinyasa: <u>From Corpse Pose **(Pg 206),** inhale and bending your elbows and expand your chest,</u> now exhale to Fish Pose, or **Hard Vinyasa: (Pg 53** / Jump Forward Part 2)

Modifications: Place a folded blanket, or small pillow under your head or place a block between your shoulder blades.

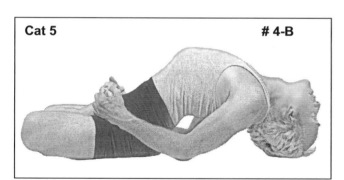

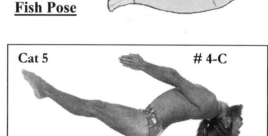

Fish Pose

CATEGORY # 6 - LEG STRETCHES (PG 147 – 166)

<u>Cat 6 / #1 - Reclining Hand-Big-Toe Pose (*Supta Padanagusthasana*):</u>

In translation, *Supta* means "supine" or "lying down," and *Pada* is "foot." The word *Angustha* means "big toe." However, I personally call this pose the Sundial Pose, because your body takes on the appearance of a sundial on the ground casting the shadow of the sun.

Benefits: Removes stiffness in the back and helps to relieve backache. This asana stretches the hamstrings and calf muscles, strengthening the knees, as it tones the hip joint and lower spine.

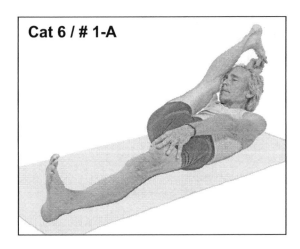

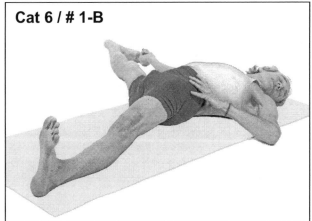

Modifications:

Keep the extended legs slightly bent, use a strap to extend your reach and use a pillow under your head, if it's more comfortable for you. When bringing the leg out to the side, you may choose to rest the thigh on a block or cushion.

Cautions:

- Asthma or bronchitis
- Stress headache
- High blood pressure
- Hip injury

If you have a sensitive back place an extra blanket on top of your yoga mat for extra support.

Vinyasa:

In Corpse Pose **(Pg 206),** inhale stretching arms overhead, then exhale into the asana.

Advanced: exit with (Vin #1 / **Pg 52**) Chakrasana.or **(easy)** roll to your side and sit up.

Instructions: (Reclining-Hand-Big-Toe-Pose – Cat 6 / # 1 / Pg 147 – 149)

1. Start from *Savanasana* **(Pg 206, photo # 1)**. Lie on your back, legs extended, feet flexed pressing out through the heels. On an exhalation draw the right knee into your chest, grasp your right, big toe with your 1st and 2nd finger and thumb on your right hand.

2. Try to straighten and extend the right leg up to the ceiling until the arms are straight keeping shoulders pressing into the floor. More flexible, bring the right leg to the torso and touch nose to the knee using your abdominals to meet the leg ½ way **(photo # 1-A).**

3. Hold for 5 breaths then, lower the right leg out to the right and bring your leg down towards the floor on your right side, as you turn your head to the left side **(photo # 1-B).** Stay in each variation for 5 breaths, and then repeat on the other side.

Cat 6 / # 2 - Western Stretch (*Paschimottanasana*):

Paschima means the "west." If you were standing, facing the east, the whole front side of your body relates to the east and the whole backside of your body relates to the west. In this posture you will stretch the whole back side of your body.

Benefits:

In the Seated Forward Bend, you will stretch and relax your muscles from the bottoms of your heels all the way up to the base of your scull. This posture stimulates nerves along your spine. The Seated Forward Bend is also used as a counter stretch for back bending postures.

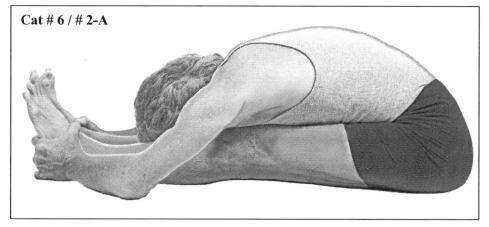
Cat # 6 / # 2-A

Cautions:
- Back injury
- Stiff neck

Modifications:
Use a strap to extend your reach. Place a folded blanket under the hips, or a small pillow under the knees. If you have short arms use a strap to reach feet.

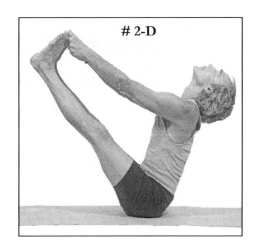

2-D

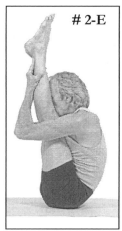

2-E

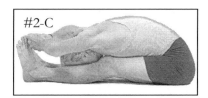

#2-C

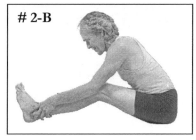

2-B

Vinyasa:

<u>**To seated position: Choose - Difficult:** (Vin # 2-B) - **(Pg 53) or Easy:** (Vin # 5) - **(Pg 57 – 58).**</u>

Into the asana – Use (Vin # 7) Eagle Wings **(Pg 59 – 60).**

Instructions: <u>**Western Stretch – Cat 6 / # 2 (Pg 149 – 150)**</u>

1. Start from The Seated Angle Position **(Pg 87, photo # 2-A),** sitting upright with your legs extended out in front of you, exhale and lower torso out over your legs, as you bend forward, placing hands on legs w /knees bent. **Beginner: stay here (photo # 2-B).**

2. **Intermediate / Adv:** Stretch further as you place chest on thighs and grab ankles with hands **(photo # 2-A),** or grasp big toes with first 2 fingers **(photo # 2-C).**

3. If you cannot grasp your toes, or ankles with your hands, just place hands on top of your legs and bend your knees slightly, or hold a strap to extend your reach.

4. **Option (# 2-D / 2-E) – Upward Facing Western Stretch:** Hold your toes and balance on buttocks, with feet upward and then hug legs and pull into chest **(photo # 2-D / 2-E).**

5. Hold each position for 5 breaths, then relax and return to Seated Angle Position.

Cat 6 / # 3 - Incline Plane (*Purvottanasana*):

Purva means the "east," relating to the whole front side of your body. In this posture you will stretch the body from under your chin to the tips of your toes.

Benefits:

In the Incline Plane, you will stretch the whole front side of your body, and strengthen your wrists, arms, and shoulders. This posture is used as the counter stretch for the Seated Forward Bend.

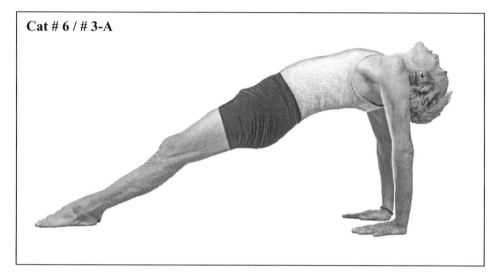

Cat # 6 / # 3-A

Cautions:

- Neck injury

- Wrist injury

- Shoulder injury

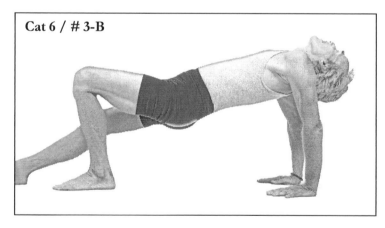

Cat 6 / # 3-B

Modifications:

Bend one or both knees, with your feet flat on the floor bringing your heels inward toward your buttocks, about a foot apart. Then push down with your hands and lift your torso upward.

Vinyasa:

Easy: In Seated Angle **(Pg 87),** Use (Vin # 7) Eagle Wings **(Pg 59-60)** to set up the asana.

Difficult: Jump into the pose from Downward Dog Pose (Vin # 2-B) - **(Pg 53-54).**

Instructions: Incline Plane – Cat 6 / # 3 (Pg 150 – 152)

1. Start from the Seated Angle Position **(Pg 87, # 2-A),** sitting up straight on the floor with your legs extended fully out in front of you and with hands on the floor, to the outside of your hips, heels of hands behind sit bones and fingers pointing toward your toes.

2. On the inhalation lift your chest, torso and hips upward, as you push hands into the floor. Ideally your legs straight, souls of feet pushing into the floor and vision upward. **Beginner:** Try bending one leg **(Pg 151, # 3-B) Adv:** go to the final pose **(photo # 3-A).**

3. When you finish, exhale, bending at the waist and lower your hips back down to the floor until you return to the Seated Angle Position.

Cat 6 / # 4 - Head Knee Pose A (*Janu Sirsasana*):

Janu means "Knee" and *Sirsa* means "Head." In this posture, from a seated position, you will bend one knee, stretching forward and placing your head down over your extended knee.

Benefits:

In the Head Knee Pose you stretch the muscles of your calf, hamstring and shoulders promoting mobility in your knee and hip joints. This pose also helps to relieve tension in your lower back, while enhancing proper function of your prostate, spleen, and kidneys.

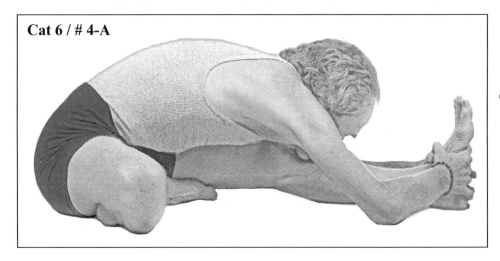

Cat 6 / # 4-A

Cautions:

- Back injury
- Knee injury

Modifications:

Bend the right knee on your extended leg and elevate, with small pillow and use a strap to extend reach. Place another support under your left knee.

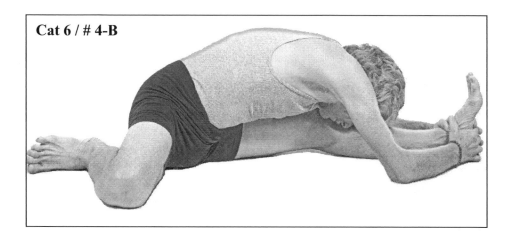

Cat 6 / # 4-B

Vinyasa: <u>Use (Vin # 7) Eagle Wings **(Pg 59 – 61).**</u>

Instructions: <u>(Head Knee Pose – Cat 6 / # 4 / Pg 152 – 153)</u>

1. From the Seated Angle **(Pg 87, - Cat 2 / #2-A),** bend your right knee, placing your right foot against your left inner thigh. Sit up straight with good posture.

2. On an inhalation, lift your arms upward, over your head, then exhale, lower your hands and torso out over the extended left leg **(photo # 4-A),** hold for 5 breaths on each side.

3. **Option (# 4-B) – Knee Bent Outward:** In this variation you will bend your right knee outward, with foot flexed **(photo # 4-B),** and again hold for 5 breaths on each side.

Cat # 6 / # 5 - Half-Bound Lotus Seated Forward Bend:

(***Ardha Baddha Padma Paschimottanasana***): The translation of *Ardha,* means "half," *Baddha,* means "bound"; *Padma* is "lotus," *Pashima* means "west." *Uttana* is an "intense stretch." This posture is a close cousin to the basic seated forward bend.

Benefits:

This posture Increases flexibility in the knees, stretches the spine, shoulders and hamstrings. Also, stimulates the liver, kidneys, ovaries, and uterus; at the same time, stretching the whole back side of your body, as you open hips and ankles.

Cautions:

Be very aware of the knees – achieving the asana at the expense of healthy knees, is a very bad trade – practice mindfully.

- Injury of back, or knees
- Weak Hips
- Stiff Ankles

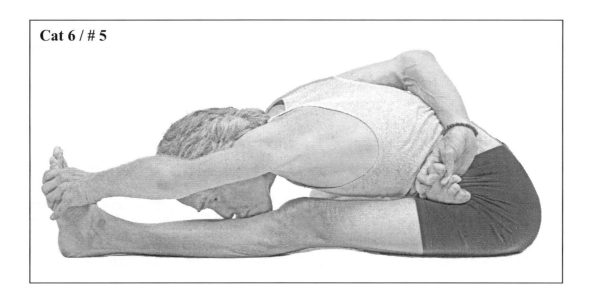

Modifications:

Bend the left knee on your extended leg and elevate with small pillow and use a strap to extend the reach behind your back. Place another support under your right knee, or choose the basic Head Knee Pose **(photo # 4-A).**

Instructions: **Half Bound Lotus Seated Forward Bend – Cat 6 / # 5 (Pg 153 – 154)**

1. From the Seated Angle **(Pg 87, Cat 2 / # 2-A),** bend your right knee, placing your right foot on top of your left thigh, in ½ lotus position.

2. Now reach your right arm behind your back and try to grasp your right toes with your right hand **(photo # 5).**

Vinyasa: <u>Choose your own path to seated- then use ½ Eagle Wings (Vin # 7) – **(Pg 59-60)**</u>

Cat 6 / # 6 - Twisted Head Knee Pose (*Parivrtta Janu Sirsasana*):

Janu means "knee" and *Sirsa* means "head." In this posture, from a seated position, you will bend one knee in as in regular Head Knee pose, only this time, twisting sideways and placing your head and torso down above your extended knee.

Benefits:

In the Twisted Head Knee Pose, you receive all the benefits of (Jana Sirsasana # I), yet with the additional stretch on the sides of your torso. This posture also places more attention to toning your spine.

Modifications:

Keep the knee slightly bent on your right extended leg and place a small elevation under your left bent knee for support. Some students find it helpful to place a folded towel under the hips.

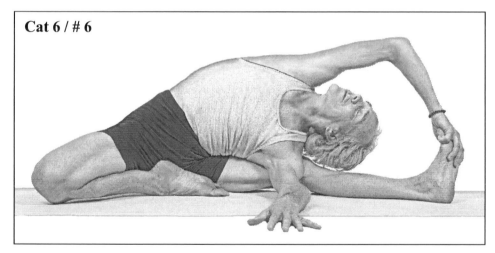

Cat 6 / # 6

Cautions:
- Back injury
- Knee injury
- Weak Hips
- Tight Ankles

Vinyasa: To seated position – **Hard:** (Vin# 2-B) Pg 53 / **Easy:** (Vin # 5) - **(Pg 57-58)**
To the pose – Inhale lift arms, then exhale to pose. (Vin # 6) between sides **(Pg 58-59)**

Instructions: Twisted Head Knee Pose – Cat 6 / # 6 (Pg 155 – 156)

1. Start the Twisted Head Knee Pose from Seated Angle Position **(Pg 87 / photo # 2-A)**, sitting up straight with your legs stretched fully out in front of you.

2. Bend your right knee, placing right foot against left inner thigh, and try to expand your legs' knees out away from one another. Then lower left shoulder over left leg.

3. In this posture, you will stretch the sides of your torso and your legs as you rotate the front of your torso upward **(photo # 6).**

4. Hold this position for 5 complete breaths on both sides.

Cat 6 / # 7 - Expanded Seated Angle (*Upavistha Konasana*):

The word *Upavistha* means "seated position," and the word *Kona* means "an angle." In this pose you will have your legs stretched outward, for this variation of Seated Angle.

Benefits:

In Expanded Seated Angle, you stretch muscles of the hamstrings, calves, and back. This posture also helps to circulate a healthy blood flow to your pelvic region and can often prevent a hernia.

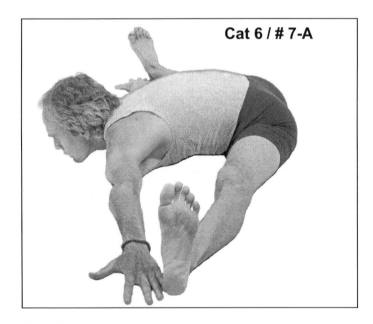

Cat 6 / # 7-A

Cautions:

- Back injury
- Knee injury
- Hip Injury
- Pregnancy

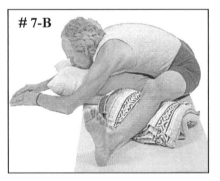

7-B

Modifications:

Keep the knees slightly bent and place a large bolster and pillow under your torso or a small block, or you could fold a blanket under your knees for support **(photo 7-B).** You can also grasp onto a strap from your hands, out around your feet.

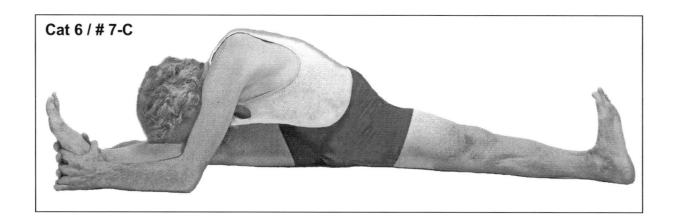

Cat 6 / # 7-C

Vinyasa: <u>From Seated Angle Pose **(Pg 87, photo #2-A)**,</u> <u>Use: Vin # 7 **(Pg 59 – 60)**</u>
<u>*Use the Eagle Wings to enter and exit each side and the middle stretch.</u>

Instructions: <u>Expanded Seated Angle – Cat 6 / # 7 (Pg 156 – 158)</u>

1. Start the Expanded Angle Posture from Seated Angle **(Pg 87 / photo #2-A),** sitting up straight with your legs stretched fully out in front of you.

2. Now stretch both legs apart from one another until you have reached your maximum comfortable and safe stretch.

3. On an exhalation, slowly hinge forward at your waist, as you try to lower your torso out over the floor in front of your hips **(photo #7-A).**

4. Less flexible - please see Modifications, or try **(Option 7-B)** with use of props.

5. Hold this position for five complete breaths, and when finished, inhale lifting your arms and torso upright and relax. Then move on to **(Option 7-C).**

6. **Option (7-C)**: Stretch to the right side. On an exhalation, gently and hinge forward at your waist, as you try to lower your torso out over your right leg **(photo #7-C).** Then repeat on the left side for 5 breaths.

When you finish, you can relax back to Seated Angle Pose, or try the additional options listed below. Hold each option for 5 breaths.

7. **Option (7-D / 7-E) – Tortoise Pose (*Kurmasana*)** – The Tortoise pose is a separate asana in itself, yet a very close relative of "Expanded Seated Angle Pose," so we will practice in this section. Follow instructions 1 and 2, then bend your knees enough to slide your arms under your knees, as you rest your torso on the floor **(photo # 7-D).** The next step is called *Supta Kurmasana* and you will try to place your feet behind your head and arms wrapped around, behind your back **(photo # 7-E).**

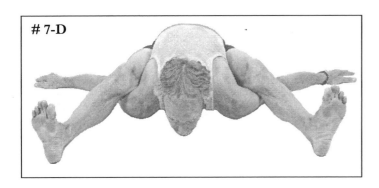 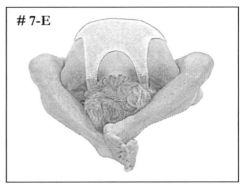

Cat 6 / # 8 - Shooting the Bow (*Akarna Dhanurasana*):

In the Sanskrit language, the preface "A" indicates the sense of "closeness," The word *Karna* means "ear," and *Dhanur* means "bow". In this posture you will resemble an archer pulling the bowstring.

Benefits:

In (Shooting the Bow Pose), you will expand your chest and hips, stretch your hamstrings, and create mobility in your knee joints. This posture also strengthens your arms and relieves tension from your low back.

Modifications:

Try - Rock the Baby **(Pg 78, Cat 1 / photo # 3)** or keep your knee slightly bent on the extended right leg and rest left foot on right thigh and use straps to grab the feet with your hands.

Cautions:

- Back injury, Neck injury and Ankle injury.

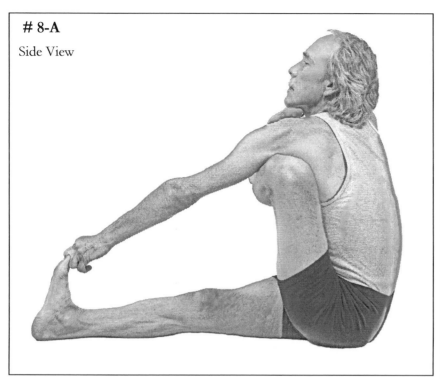

8-A
Side View

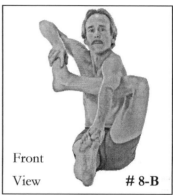

Front
View   # 8-B

Vinyasa:

Choose from: **Easy-** Vin # 5 **(Pg 57 – 58),** Missing Link- Vin #4 (Pg #57, 58), or **Difficult**- Vin # 2-B **(Pg 53).**

Instructions: <u>**Shooting the Bow – Cat 6 / # 8 (Pg 158 – 159)**</u>

1. Start Shooting the Bow pose from the Seated Angle **(Pg 87, Cat 2 / # 2-A),** sitting up straight with your legs fully stretched out in front of you.

2. Place your left foot on top of your right thigh, and try to hold your left ankle with your right hand as you lift your ankle up off your thigh.

3. Now reach forward with your left hand and try to take hold of your right toes – see **(Photo # 8-A, 8-B).** Hold this position for five complete breaths.

4. When finished exhale, as you release the grip on your toes and relax into seated angle pose, then repeat the same exercise on the opposite side.

5. **Modification:** bend your extended right leg and rest your left foot on your right thigh.

Cat 6 / # 9 - Heron Pose (*Krunchasana*):

In translation *Krunch,* means "heron," which is a large wading bird common near the shores of open water and in wetlands over most of North America and Central America. In this pose, you will resemble the posture of a heron.

Benefits:

In the Heron, you will stretch your back, hips, and hamstrings, as you stimulate your heart and abdominal organs.

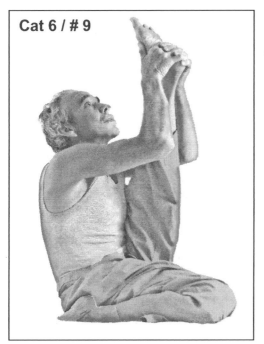

Cat 6 / # 9

Cautions:

- Menstruation

- Knee injury

- Ankle problems

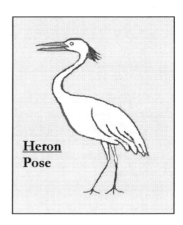

Heron Pose

Modifications:

Keep the knee slightly bent on the raised leg and sit on a block. Some students like to place their raised leg on the wall.

Vinyasa:

Choose from: **Hard-** Vin # 2-B **(Pg 53); Easy-** Vin # 5 **(Pg 57)** or Vin # 6 **(Pg 58)**

Instructions: Heron Pose – Cat 6 / # 9 (Pg 160 – 161)

1. Start in Seated Angle Pose **(Pg 87 / photo # 2-A).** Bend your right knee, with ankle on the outside of your right thigh muscle. Then bend your left knee, placing the left foot flat on the floor, just in front of the left sit bone.

2. Now grasp the left foot with both hands and try to lift your left leg up in front of your torso. Lean back slightly, but keep the front torso long **(photo # 9)**. Hold this position for 5 breaths then slowly and mindfully straighten your legs and repeat on the opposite side.

Cat 6 / # 10 - Sage Pose (*Marichyasana* A):

Marichi is the great-grandfather of Manu "man, thinking, intelligent," the Vedic Adam, and the "father" of humanity. *Marichi* literally means "a ray of light," and in this asana you will inspire positive thinking and light.

Benefits:

This asana sequence is said to calm the brain, as you stretch arms, shoulders, ankles, and spine. In addition, you will help to stimulate the liver, and the kidneys will improve digestion.

Modifications: Sit on a block or a thick blanket and place a folded blanket under the knee of the extended leg. To extend your reach, you may use straps for binding.

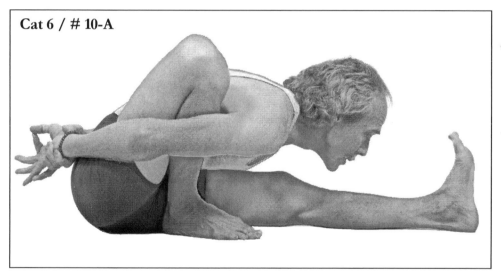

Cat 6 / # 10-A

Cautions:

- Stiff ankles
- Knee injury
- Back Injury

This asana is often practiced with its (Other 3 variations) for a balanced approach. After you complete the base pose try the other 3-options listed in the instructions on **(Pg 162).**

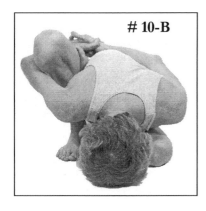

10-B

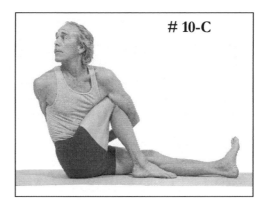

10-C

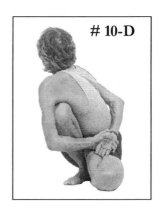

10-D

Vinyasa:

Choose from: **Hard-** Vin # 2-B **(Pg 53); Easy-** Vin # 5 **(Pg 57)**, Vin # 6 **(Pg 58)**

Instructions: **Sage Pose – Cat 6 / # 10 (Pg 161 – 162)**

1. Start in **Seated Angle (Pg 87 - Cat 2 / # 2-A).** Bend your right knee and place the foot on the floor, with the heel as close to the left sitting bone as possible. Keep the left leg extended and rotated, slightly inward, with foot flexed and toes pointing upward.

2. Try to place the inner right thigh firmly against the right side of the torso and rib cage. Now wrap your right arm around the outside of your right knee, and try to grab your wrist behind your back **(# 10-A).**

3. **Option (# 10-B) – Half Lotus:** Follow the same instructions as for *Marichyasana* A, only this time, you will place your left foot in ½ lotus on top of your right thigh, as you bend forward at the waist and drop your head toward the floor.

4. Now try to wrap your right arm around the outside of your right knee, and try to grab your left wrist behind your back **(# 10-B).**

5. **Option (# 10-C) – Sage Bound Twist:** Follow the same instructions as for *Marichyasana* A, only this time you will twist your torso to the right and wrap your left arm around your right bent knee, as you grasp your right wrist behind your back with your left hand **(photo # 10-C).**

6. **Option (# 10-D) – Twisted Half Lotus Bind:** Follow the same instructions as you did for **(10-B)**, only instead of bending forward at the waist. This time you will twist to the right and bind your left arm around your right bent knee, as you try to sit up tall and twist to your right.

Cat 6 / # 11 - One Leg Behind-Head (*Eka Pada Sirsasana*):

The word *Eka* means "one" and *Pada* means "foot". In this advanced yoga pose, you will place one foot or leg behind your head.

Benefits:

Helps to develop supple legs, hips and knees; although don't allow your ego to lead you to an injury – practice mindfully.

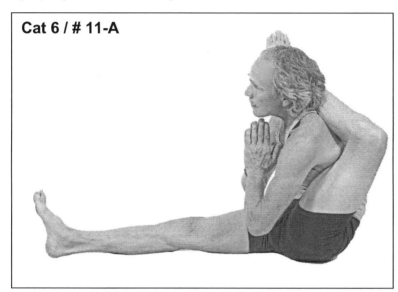

Cat 6 / # 11-A

Cautions:

- Neck injury
- Back injury
- Hip injury
- Knee injury

(Be very careful)

Vinyasa: Hard- Vin # 2-B **(Pg 53)**; Easy- Vin # 5 **(Pg 57)** or Vin # 6 **(Pg 58)**

Modifications: Try Rock the Baby pose **(Pg 78 Photo # 3)** or Shooting the Bow pose **(Pg 158, Photo #8)**, or as option, or do not commit to placing the leg behind the head, just go part way.

Instructions: **One Leg Behind Head / Options – Cat 6 / # 11 (Pg 163 – 164)**

1. From a seated position in Seated Angle / **(Pg 87, Cat 2 / # 2-A)**, cradle your left leg like you are rocking a baby (back and forth), this is a great warm-up exercise.

2. Slowly and mindfully bring your bent left leg up toward your head. Now using awareness, and *if* you have the flexibility, place your left leg behind your head **(Cat 6, # 11-A)**. Hold this position for 5 breaths on each side, and remember to exit the pose slowly and mindfully.

3. **Option 11-B - Full Standing Position:** From **(photo 11-A),** Place your hands on your right thigh and try to take a full standing position. Hold for 5 breaths on each side.

4. **Option 11-C - Lift up On Arms:** From **(photo 11-A),** Put hands on the ground, as you lift your hips off the floor and gaze upward.

5. **Option 11-D** – Lie down on the floor with both legs behind your head, hands over your heart, and hold for 5 breaths. When finished, exit mindfully to avoid injury.

Box ready A, B, C

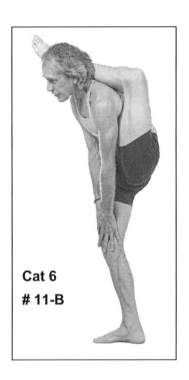

Cat 6
11-B

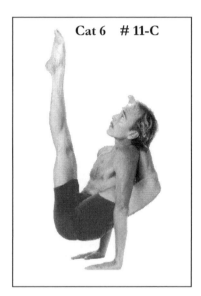

Cat 6   # 11-C

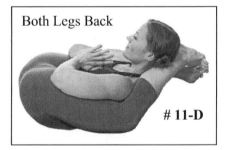

From Cat 6 # 11-A
Lie on your back and place both legs behind your head.
Hold for 5 breaths see photo
11-D – Sara Turk (Demo)

Both Legs Back

11-D

Cat 6 / # 12 - Monkey Pose (*Hanumanasana*):

The Sanskrit name for "Monkey Pose" is *Hanumanasana* and is named after the Hindu monkey god, *Hanuman*. In an ancient story, *Hanuman* took one big giant leap all the way from India to Sri Lanka, and then one more leap to return to India. The Monkey Pose reflects his leap.

The Monkey Pose, is commonly known as "the splits," and is considered to be an advanced leg stretch and hip-opener. The yoga version of this pose keeps the hips squared to the front, different than the version practiced in dance where the hips are opened more to the side.

- **Cautions:** Injury to Groin, Back Hips or Knees.

Benefits:

The Monkey Pose will open the hamstrings, quadriceps, groin, and hip flexors, as it tones and stimulates the abdominal organs. This pose also simultaneously stretches the front and back of your legs. Regularly practicing will help to keep your legs and hips supple, which can help prevent injury in other activities.

Modifications:

Try placing a yoga block under each hand to help support yourself and to help bring your torso more upright. Another nice modification is to place a block underneath your hamstring for support, or place a folded, firm blanket or a yoga bolster beneath your pelvis for support.

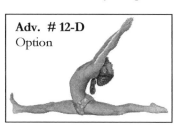

Adv. # 12-D
Option

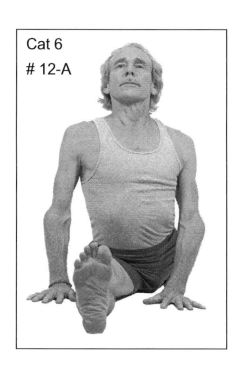

Cat 6
12-A

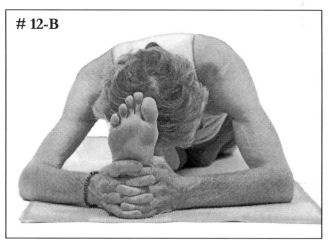

12-B

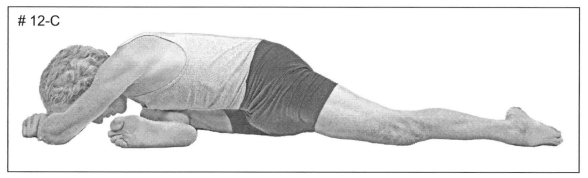

12-C

Vinyasa: Your choice to Seated or use Eagle Wings-Vin # 6 **(Pg 59-60**) into the pose.

Instructions: <u>Monkey Pose – Cat 6 / # 12 / Pg 164 – 166</u>

1. Start from Downward Facing Dog Pose **(Pg 190 photo # 3-A):** then step slowly forward with your right leg, allowing your hips to move toward the floor.

2. Keep your right heel on the floor and lean your torso slightly forward, as you press your fingertips firmly on the floor. You could also place your hands onto yoga blocks, set alongside each hip.

3. Straighten your right leg, but do not lock or hyperextend your knee. Try to keep your hips squared to the front of your yoga mat and parallel to one another. Check behind you, and try to keep your left leg reaching directly behind you and not off to the side.

4. **Option (12-A) - Monkey Torso Up:** Try to keep your torso upright, which also creates more of a back stretch. Modify by placing a block under your right hamstring muscle. Hold for 5 breaths.

5. **Option (12-B) – Monkey Forward Fold:** From **(12-A):** Fold your torso forward out over the extended leg and strive to bring your torso toward your thigh. Modify by bending the extended leg slightly and placing a block under your right hamstring muscle. Hold for 5 breaths.

6. **Option (12-C) – Pigeon Pose (Kapotasana):** From **(12-A):** now bend the right knee to about 90 degrees, as you lean forward and feel the hip opening. Modify by placing a block or folded blanket under hips, or under your right hamstring muscle.

7. **Option (12-D) – Full Monkey Pose:** Lift arms up over your head and arch backward, being mindful to keep hips squared to the front wall.

CATEGORY # 7 – BACK BEND POSTURES (PG 166 – 181)

<u>Cat 7 / # 1 - Cobra Pose (*Bhujangasana*):</u>

Cobra Pose in Sanskrit is *Bhujangasana,* which means "serpent" or a "cobra snake." In this asana you will take on the appearance and energy of a cobra snake as it slowly uncoils, lifting its head and torso up into the air. Cobra is a beginning backbend that will help to prepare your body for deeper backbends.

Benefits:
Cobra Pose will increase the flexibility of the spine as it stretches the chest, while strengthening the spine and shoulders. This pose also stimulates the abdominal organs, improving digestion

and as an energizing backbend, Cobra reduces stress and fatigue. In addition, Cobra firms and tones the shoulders, abdomen, and buttocks.

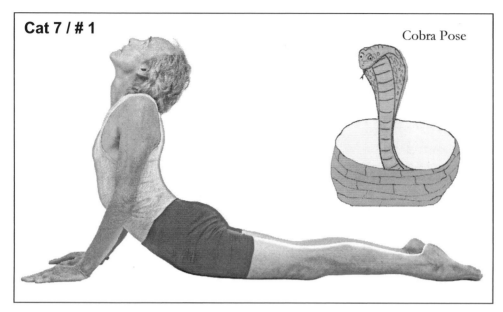

Cat 7 / # 1

Cobra Pose

Cautions:

- Carpal tunnel
- Back injury
- Wrist injury
- Pregnancy

Modifications:

If you are less flexible you can benefit from practicing Cobra while standing facing a wall, with your hands placed against the wall. Another modification is to keep your arms bent, resting on your elbows in Sphinx Pose and move your feet wider apart.

Vinyasa:
Choose: Soft- Easy Breezy -Vin # 6 **(Pg 58) Moderate**: take 'Up Dog' to 'Down Dog' then relax into Cobra Pose.

Instructions: Cobra Pose – Cat 7 / # 1 (Pg 166 – 168)

1. Begin by lying face-down on the floor with your legs extended behind you, spread a few inches apart. The tops of your feet should rest on the mat — do not tuck your toes, as this can crunch your spine.

2. Place your hands under your shoulders with your fingers pointing toward the top of the mat. Press down through the tops of your feet and your pubic bone, and spread your toes.

3. Inhale as you gently lift your head and chest off the floor. Keep your thighs on the floor.

4. Draw your shoulders back and lift your heart forward, but avoid crunching your neck. Keep your shoulders dropped away from your ears **(photo # 1)**.

5. Hold this position for 5 breaths, or longer, then relax back to the floor in Childs Pose, or move on through to vinyasa.

Cat 7 /# 2 - Upward Facing Dog (*Urdhva Mukha Svanasana*):

Urdva Mukha means "upward facing" and *Svana* relates to a "dog." In this posture, you will resemble a dog stretching upward as it lengthens its legs and back after a nice nap. This is a very common asana, used in many styles as an asana, or part of a vinyasa.

Benefits:

Upward-Facing Dog stretches and creates flexibility in the spine and chest, as it strengthens the wrists, arms, and shoulders. By strengthening and expanding the upper body and chest it improves posture. In addition, this asana tones the torso's back and abdomen, which stimulates the abdominal organs, and improves digestion, as it firms buttocks and thighs.

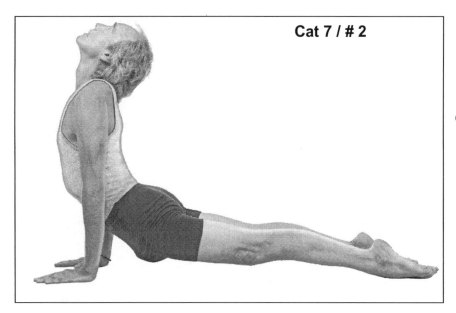

Cat 7 / # 2

Cautions:
- Carpal tunnel
- Back injury
- Wrist injury
- Pregnancy

Modifications:

Place a pillow or bolster up under your thighs and try moving feet further apart. Another option is to practice Cobra pose until you gain flexibility and strength.

Vinyasa:

Inhale to enter, then exhale to exit. This works from Down Dog **(Pg 190)** or Child's Pose **(Pg 94)** Or Staff Pose **(Pg 187).**

Instructions: Upward Facing Dog – Cat 7 / # 2 (Pg 168 – 169)

1. Start by lying face-down on the floor, with your legs extended behind you, and spread a few inches apart. The tops of your feet should rest on your yoga mat with toes pointed.

2. Place your hands on the floor beside your torso, next to your lower ribs. Point your fingers forward and keep elbows in close to your ribcage.

3. Inhale as you press through your hands and straighten your arms, expand our chest and lift your torso and your upper legs a few inches off the floor. Try to keep your shoulders back, but don't crunch the neck – lift up through the spine **(photo # 2).**

4. Hold this pose for 5 breaths. To release, exhale as you slowly lower your torso and forehead to your mat, then Relax to Child's Pose, or move into a vinyasa.

Cat 7 / # 3 - Locust Pose (*Salabhasana*) & Half Locust:

Ardha means "Half" and *Salabha* means the insect called a "locust." In this posture, you will feel the energy of the Earth, as you rest your stomach on the ground, much like a locust resting in the grass.

Benefits:

Salabhasana strengthens and increases flexibility throughout the entire back side of the body, which includes the spine, legs, buttocks, and all of the muscles along-side the ribs and upper torso. Strengthening upper back muscles improves posture and helps relieve stress and fatigue.

This asana also tones the abdominal muscles and the chest which stimulates your abdominal organs and aids in digestion.

Modifications:

Place your arms and hands underneath your torso and lift only one leg off the mat. You will really stretch under your chin in this asana, to assist, place a blanket up under your chest to create a few inches of elevation, this will take any pressure off your neck.

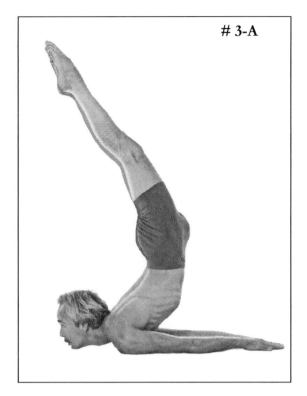

 # 3-A

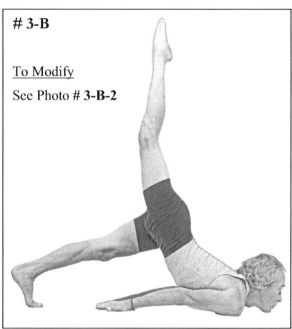

 # 3-B

<u>To Modify</u>
See Photo **# 3-B-2**

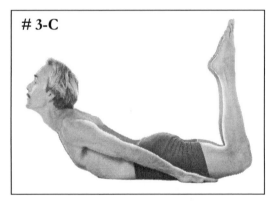

 # 3-C

 # 3-D

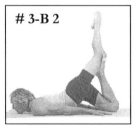

 # 3-B 2

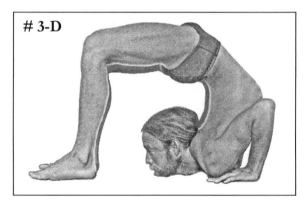

Cautions:

- Injury to neck
- Sensitive Chest
- Pregnancy

<u>Option # 3-B-2</u>
Bend right knee
and rest left leg on
your foot. Hold for
5 breaths.

Vinyasa: <u>Cobra **(Pg 166),** then exhale to Down Dog **(Pg 190),** then rest on your stomach for</u> <u>Locust Pose. Now expand your chest and arch your back, using your core muscles as you lift</u> <u>your legs upward.</u>

Instructions: <u>Locust Pose – Cat 7 / # 3 (Pg 169 – 171)</u>

1. Lie down on your stomach with your arms extended by your sides, and palms facing downward. Turn your head forward, while resting your chin on the floor.

2. Place your hands up under your thighs, palms facing downward as you stretch your chin out long, as though you are trying to look out in front of you.

3. Lift knees, hips and chest off the floor. This is **Full Locust Pose (photo # 3-A).**

4. **Option (3-B) Half Locust Pose:** Follow Instructions 1 and 2 on an inhalation' lift your right leg backward and upward, pressing down with your left leg and foot into the floor **(Photo #3-B).** To modify – place a folded blanket under your chest, to take pressure off your neck. Hold for 5 breaths on each side. **As an option (photo # 3-B-2).**

5. **Option (3-C) Grounded Full Locust:** Rest on stomach with knees bent, resting arms by your sides, with palms facing downward. Now expand your chest and arch your back, as you lift your knees and shoulders off the floor **(Photo # 3-C).** Hold for 5 breaths.

6. **Option (3-D) Flying Locust / Feet to Floor – Advanced:** From **(photo 3-A)** bend your knees and lower your feet toward your head and then rest feet on the floor, as you relax and breath **(photo # 3-D). (Be very careful and mindful – you can injure your back and neck in this asana).**

Cat 7 / # 4 - Bow (Dhanurasana:

In Sanskrit language, *Dhanur* means "bow" and in this posture you will form an arched bow with your body; your arms acting as the bowstring, as you hold onto your ankles.

Benefits:

This posture helps to tone abdominal muscles, and with regular practice, assist in creating a very elastic spine. You will also open your shoulders, as you stretch your thighs and expand your chest. This is a good pose to help over-come bad posture and can assist with correcting spinal alignment. Additionally, it tones abdominals, quadriceps, ankles, and hip flexors.

Cautions: Blood pressure Problem, Pregnancy or Back injury.

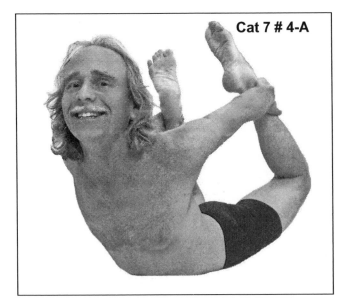
Cat 7 # 4-A

Modifications:

Extend your reach, using a yoga strap to grasp ankles, or keep knees further apart. If you do not yet have the flexibility to perform Bow Pose, try Half Bow by simply grasping one ankle with one hand.

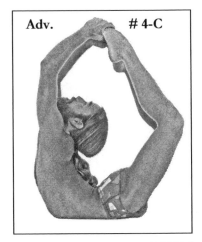
Adv.   # 4-C

Advanced – Grasp toes instead of ankles and lift

Feet and hands up over your head – as you gaze upward **(Photo # 4-C)**

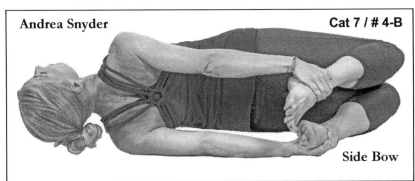
Andrea Snyder   Cat 7 / # 4-B

Side Bow

Vinyasa: Easy Breezy-Vin # 6 **(Pg 58)** or take Cobra **(Pg 166)** or Up Dog **(Pg 168)**

Then to Down Dog **(Pg 190)** or Child's pose **(Pg 94)** – now move into Bow Pose.

Instructions: Bow Pose – Cat 7 / # 4 (Pg 171 – 173)

1. Start by lying flat on your stomach with your chin on your mat and hands resting by your sides.

2. Bring your heels as close to your buttocks as you can, keeping your knees hips-width apart. Now reach back with both hands and grab hold of your ankles.

3. On an inhalation, lift your ankles up toward the ceiling, drawing your thighs up and off your yoga mat. Lifting your head, expanding your chest, and lift shoulders off the mat **(photo # 4-A).**

4. Gaze forward and upward holding this pose for 5 breaths. When finished slowly release your ankles and return to the floor. Or you may move into Side Bow **(photo # 4-B)**.

5. **Option (4-B) Side Bow (*Parsva Dhanurasana*):** Practice steps 1-4, as listed above for the Bow Pose. Then exhale, and bring your left shoulder to the floor, rolling over to your left side until you are lying completely on your left side **(photo # 4-B).** Hold for up to 5 breaths on each side.

6. **Option (4-C) Advanced Bow** / see photo and instructions **(Pg 172, # 4-C).**

Cat 7 / # 5 - Camel Posture (*Ustrasana*):

Ustra means "Camel." In this backward arching posture, you will somewhat resemble the hump on a camel's back.

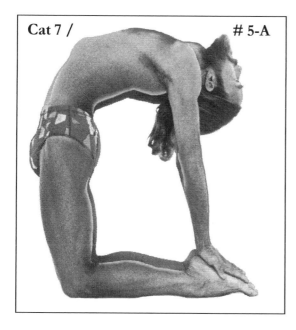

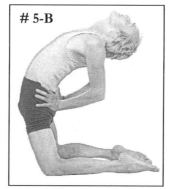

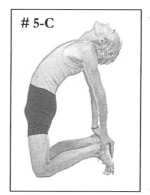

Cautions:

- High Blood pressure
- Headaches
- Back injury
- Neck injury

Benefits:

The Camel pose stretches the front of the body, the chest, abdomen, quadriceps, and hip flexors. At the same time improves spinal flexibility, while also strengthening your back muscles and improving posture. This asana creates space in the chest and lungs, helping to increase breathing capacity. Camel pose also stimulates the kidneys, which improves digestion.

Modifications:

These simple modifications will assist you in comfortability when practicing Camel Pose.

Place a folded towel under your knees and blocks under your hands, or try placing hands on top of your heels, with feet flexed. If you have neck issues, do not drop head back.

Vinyasa:

Use Missing Link-Vin #5 - **(Pg 55)** steps 1–3, then exhale into Camel Pose **(Pg 173).**

Instructions: <u>Camel Pose – Cat 7 / # 5 / (Pg 173 – 174)</u>

1. Begin in Thunder Bolt Pose **(Pg 92, photo # 6).** Then move your knees hip-width apart, as you lift your buttocks up off your heels.
2. Now exhale and expand your chest, as you arch backward, placing your hands onto your feet, or ankles **(photo # 5-A).** To Modify – Place hands on blocks.
3. Keep your thighs perpendicular to the floor, with your hips up over your knees and resting hands on the soles of your feet.
4. **Option (5-B) Hands on Hips:** For an easier version, place your hands on your hips pushing hips forward and downward as you arch backward **(photo # 5-B).**
5. **Option (5-C) Hands on Heels:** With Flexed feet, place your hands on your heels. **(Photo # 5-C).**
6. Hold for 5 breaths, then return to Thunder Bolt Pose, or move though a vinyasa.

<u>Cat 7 / # 6 - Pigeon Pose (*Kapotasana*):</u>

The word *Kapota* means "pigeon" and *Asana* means "pose." In this asana you will puff your chest out like a proud pigeon. There are several other poses which come by the same name. This pose is technically a different and yet very closely related to the Camel Pose. Many students practice this asana as an extension or 2nd step of the Camel Pose.

Benefits:

This asana stretches the front side of the body, ankles, thighs and groins, in addition to abdomen, chest, and throat. This pose tones hip flexors (psoas), and strengthens back muscles for improved posture.

This version of Pigeon will also stimulate the organs of the abdomen and neck.

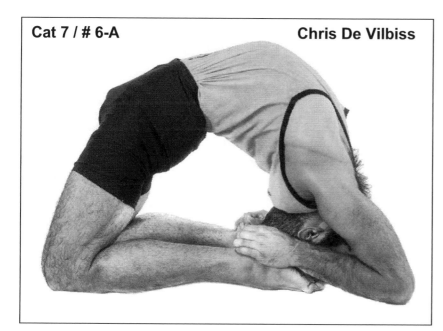

Cat 7 / # 6-A   Chris De Vilbiss

Cautions:

- Blood pressure issue
- Migraine
- Insomnia
- Back injury
- Neck injury

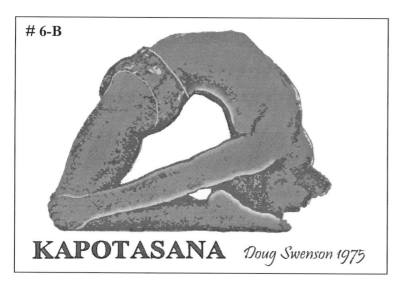

6-B

KAPOTASANA   *Doug Swenson 1975*

Above - Chris De VilBiss

Holding ankles, with elbows on floor **(Option 5-A).**

Doug Swenson (Photo Art)

The same pose, with different hand and arm placement **(Option 6-B).**

Modifications:

From Camel Pose **(Cat 7 # 5-A, Pg 173): Beginner** – lay back on the floor with bent knees and a bolster under your spine to create the arched back as you relax for 5 breaths. You can also reach your arms up over your head with elbows bent, to further stretch your triceps. **Intermediate** – practice Camel Pose with your back to the wall and toes touching the wall, then lean back and place hands on the wall as you arch and expend your chest.

Vinyasa:

<u>**Soft:**</u> use Vin # 6 **(Pg 58-59);** <u>**Hard:**</u> take Up-dog to Down-dog, then move into the pose.

Instructions: <u>**Pigeon Pose – Cat 7 / # 6 (Pg 174 – 176)**</u>

1. **Advanced:** Begin in Camel Pose **(Pg 173 - photo # 5-B),** now exhale and expand your chest, as you arch backward, and do a backbend from your knees.

2. Keep your hands up over your head, with elbows bent, as you try grabbing your feet or ankles with your hands **(photo # 6-A).**

3. **Option (photo # 6-B) – Hands on Knees:** Follow the first instruction, then place your hands on your thighs, down as close to the knees as possible.

4. From here, deepen the back bend while holding onto the knees or thighs, as you lower your head to the souls of your feet **(photo # 6-B).**

5. Hold for 5 breaths, then inhale and slowly return to Camel – then exhale and rest for a few breaths in Child's Pose, with torso on your thighs and arms extended forward.

<u>Cat 7 / # 7 - Upside Down Bow (*Urdhva Dhanurasana*):</u>

In Sanskrit, the word *Urdhva* means "upward" and *Dhanu* relates to a "bow." In this posture, you will form an upside down-bow. In America, this posture is often called the Wheel Posture, or Back Bend.

Benefits:

Upside Down Bow & Back Bend postures are excellent for creating a supple spine, expanding your chest and strengthening your arms and wrist. This upside down posture also helps to send oxygenated blood to your brain, leaving you with a very relaxed and refreshed feeling.

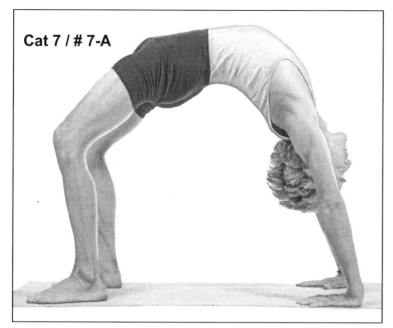

Cat 7 / # 7-A

Cautions:

- Back, Neck injury
- Neck injury
- Eye injury
- Wrist Injury

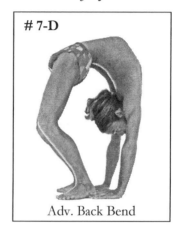

7-D

Adv. Back Bend

Modifications:

For an easier variation, try Bridge Pose **(Pg 144, photo # 3-A, B).** Full backbend option: place a pair of blocks under your hands, with the blocks at the base of the wall. The third option is to refrain from the full backbend and simply go part way and rest on your head.

Vinyasa:

Soft: use Vin # 6 **(Pg 58 – 59); Hard:** take Up-dog to Down-dog, then move into the pose.

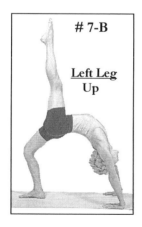

7-B

Left Leg Up

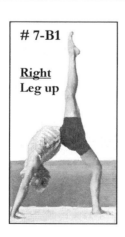

7-B1

Right Leg up

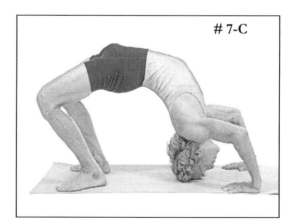

7-C

Instructions: Upside Down Bow – Cat 7 / # 7 (Pg 176 – 178)

1. Start from the Corpse Pose **(Pg 206, photo # 1)** lie on the ground, extend your arms by your sides, palms facing up-ward your feet should be about one foot apart.

2. Bend your knees and draw your feet up toward your hips, keeping your feet flat on the ground, as you place your hands on the floor beside your ears. Tuck your hands, palms down, under shoulders. **Beginners stay here – or only lift hips. Not shoulders.**

3. **Intermediate:** Inhale, as you push down with your hands and feet, trying to lift your torso up to rest on top of your head **(photo # 7-C).**

4. **Advanced:** Continue on to pushing up with your hands and feet. Straighten your elbows and raise your hips until your body forms a large arch or wheel **(photo # 7-A).**

5. **Option (# 7-B):** Lift One Leg Straight Upward and hold for 5 breaths on each side.

6. **Option (# 7-D):** Very flexible students try this variation for a greater stretch. When finished lower your torso down and relax your whole body back into Corpse Pose.

Back Bend Counter stretch -

After Back bends, it is best to counter stretch, with: Happy Baby **(Pg 103 - # 15),** or Child's Pose **(Pg 94, photo # 8),** or Supine Twist **(Pg 182, photo # 1).**

Cat 7 / # 8 - One-Leg King Pigeon Pose (*Eka Pada Rajakapotasana*):

In the Sanskrit language *Eka* means "one," *Pada* Means "foot," *Raja* means "king" and *kapota* means "pigeon." Then *asana* means "pose." In this asana, you will expand and puff your chest up like a proud pigeon.

Benefits:

In Pigeon Pose, you will stretch thighs, groins, and abdomen. It can also be felt in specific upper-leg and hip muscles, including the psoas and piriformis. This pose relieves tension in the chest and shoulders, and it also stimulates the abdominal organs, which can help to regulate digestion.

Modifications:

Use a strap to extend reach, or practice with Left bent leg on a wall behind you.

Vinyasa:

<u>Soft:</u> use Vin # 6 **(Pg 58, 59); Hard:** take Up-dog to Down-dog, then move to pose.

Cat 7 / # 8-A

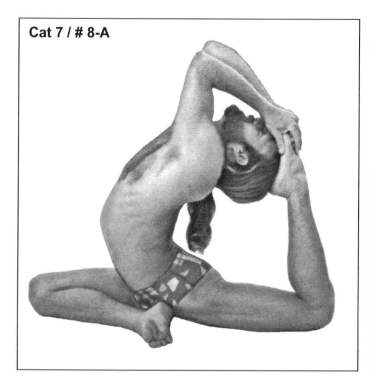

Cautions:

- Ankle injury
- Knee injury
- Back problems
- Pregnancy

 # 8-B

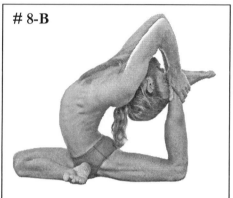

Instructions: <u>**One Leg King Pigeon – Cat 7 / # 8 (Pg 178 – 179)**</u>

1. Start in Down Dog Pose **(Pg 190, photo # 3-A).**

2. Then bring your right knee up to rest on the floor between your hands, placing your right ankle near your left wrist. Extend your left leg behind you, so your kneecap and the top of your foot rest on the floor.

3. Push down through your fingertips as you lift your torso away from your thigh. Lengthen the front of your body. Release your tailbone back toward your heels. Work on squaring your hips to the front of our mat.

4. Expand our chest and arch your back. **Beginners – Intermediate:** Stay here with hands on the floor under your shoulders - hold for 5 breaths.

5. **Intermediate – Advanced**: grab your left foot with your left hand and lift up toward the back of your head. Hold your foot with both hands, elbows 1-foot apart, then drop head back with sole of foot resting on top of your head, or beyond **(photo # 8-A / 8-B).**

6. Hold for 5 breaths on each side, then slowly release to Child's Pose **(Pg 93, photo # 8)** or take a vinyasa.

Cat 7 / # 9 - Frog Pose (*Ardha Bhekasana*) and Half Frog -

The name comes from the Sanskrit words: *Ardha* meaning "half" and *Bheka* meaning "frog" and the word *asana* meaning "posture." In this pose, you will resemble a frog resting on the shore of a quiet pond.

Benefits:

This yoga asana will tone your hips and buttocks, stretch and open your groins and your thighs. In addition, this pose will inspire more flexibility in your spine, legs, back muscles, and knees.

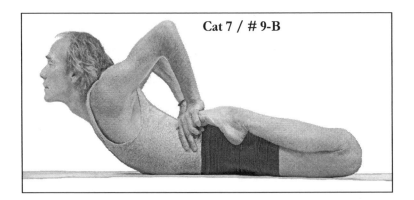

Cat 7 / # 9-B

> **This is the Full Frog pose**

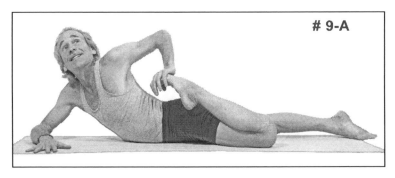

9-A

> **This is the half Frog pose**

Cautions: Injury of Knee, Hip, Shoulder and Ankle. Also Pregnancy

Vinyasa: Soft: use Vin # 6 **(Pg 58, 59); Hard**: take Up-dog to Down-dog, then move to pose.

Modifications:

Support the lift of the upper torso with a small pillow under lower ribs, and press your forearm on the floor in front of the pillow. It's best to practice ½ Frog pose, before the full variation.

Instructions: Frog Pose – Cat 7 / # 9 (Pg 180 – 181)

1. Lie on your stomach – placing right forearm on the floor parallel to the front of your mat. Then twist your torso to your left and place your left hand on top of your left foot.

2. Try to slowly rotate your left elbow toward the ceiling, slide your fingers over on top of the left foot and curl fingers over the toes. The base of your palm should be pressing the top of the foot **Half Frog Pose (photo # 9-A)** Hold for 5 breaths on each side.

3. **Option: Full Frog Pose (# 9-B)** Follow the same instructions for ½ Frog pose, only this time, strive to gasp hold of both feet at the same time – pushing both feet to the outside of the buttocks.

4. Inhale and lift your chest as high as you can, squeezing your shoulders towards one another. The higher you lift your chest, the easier it will be for you to hold your feet down **(photo # 9-B). This is the Full Frog Pose**

5. Maintain this posture until five breaths and then slowly release to the ground and relax.

CATEGORY # 8 - TWISTING POSTURES (PG 181 – 187)

Cat 8 / # 1 - Supine Twist (*Supta Matsyendrasana*):

In *Sanskrit*, the pose is called "*Supta Matsyendrasana*." This pose is named after an "ancient yoga deity," or *siddhi*, called *Matseyendra*. The name *Matseyendra* literally means "lord of the fishes," this pose is sometimes referred to as Reclined Lord of the Fishes Pose. It is the supine (lying-down) version of the popular seated twist.

The Supine Twist is easy to practice, and a wonderful way to tone your spine and release tension in your back. It's especially helpful after practicing yoga back bends, or forward bends, to create a soothing balance.

Benefits:

The Supine Twist will invigorate your entire spine with a gentle twisting that stretches the muscles in your back and hips. Be sure to combine this exercise with yoga breathing techniques.

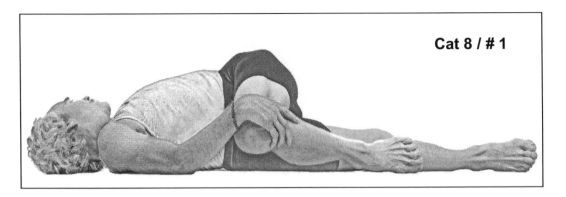

Cat 8 / # 1

Modifications:

Try resting your left knee and leg on a bolster, a firm pillow or block, and then place another folded blanket behind your back to create support on both sides. If you are more flexible, then you can choose not to use the elevation under your left knee.

Cautions: Injury of back, knee, or hip and precautions for Pregnancy.

Vinyasa: Exhale, release and with knees bent and feet flat, try the wind-shield-wiper by gently rocking hips from right to left. Then practice the pose on the opposite side for 5 breaths.

Instructions: Supine Twist – Cat 8 / # 1 (Pg 181 – 182)

1. From Corpse Pose **(Pg 206, photo # 1),** Extend your arms straight out from your shoulders, at a 90-degree angle from your torso.

2. Bend your left knee, as you try to move your left knee to the floor on the right side of your right leg. Then place your right hand on top of your left knee.

3. At the same time try to keep your shoulder flat on the floor and turn your head to the left, **(photo # 1).** Hold for 5 breaths on each side then relax back to Sponge Pose.

Cat 8 / # 2 - Twist Pose (*Ardha Matsyendrasana*):

In Hindu legend, *Matsyendra* was a "fish" which twisted around in order to hear the secrets of Yoga from Lord *Siva*. *Matsyendra* was then incarnated into human form, in order to spread the knowledge of Yoga. This posture is dedicated to *Matsyendra*, the "twisted fish." In *Sanskrit* the word *ardha*, or "half," refers to the basic twist, the full twist is practiced in Lotus.

Its Sanskrit name, "*Ardha Matsyendrasana*" is derived from four words – *ardha* means "half" and *matsya* means "fish." Then *indra* means "ruler" and *asana* means "pose."

Benefits:

Stretches shoulders, hips, neck, and spine, and helps relieve fatigue, backache, and sciatica. Fish pose also stimulates digestion and metabolism, tones kidneys and liver, and inspires relief from menstrual discomfort.

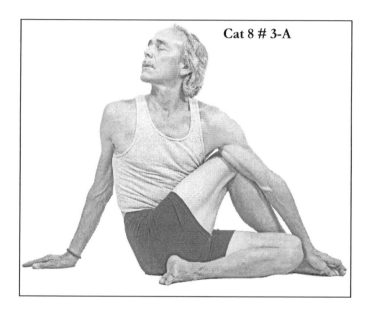

Cat 8 # 3-A

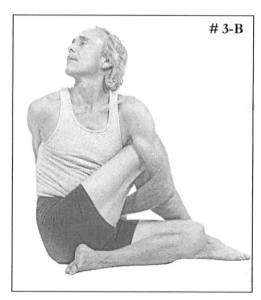

3-B

Modifications:

If it is difficult for you to place your left elbow to the outside of your right knee, bend your left arm and hug the right knee with your left arm. Many will choose to elevate the hips on a small block, or a folded blanket. Another assist is to keep the left leg straight instead of bent.

Cautions: Injury of Knees, Hips, Back and Neck.

Vinyasa: <u>Inhale twist away from the pose – then exhale move into the pose.</u>

Between sides: Vin # 6 **(Pg 58)**, or Up-dog **(Pg 168)**, or Cobra to Down-dog to Child's Pose.

Instructions: <u>Seated Twist Pose – Cat 8 / # 2 (Pg 182 – 184)</u>

1. Begin seated on the floor in Seated Angle Pose **(Pg 87 - photo # 2-A),** with your legs extended in front of you, arms resting at your sides.

2. Bend your right knee and place your right foot on floor, to the left side of your left thigh.

3. Then, lean to your left and bend your extended left leg, with the left heel coming to rest alongside your right buttocks.

4. Twist your torso to the right and gently fold your left arm around the outside of your right knee. **Less flexible, stay here for gentle twist** & Hold for 5 breaths on each side.

5. **Option (photo # 3-A):** To deepen the stretch, lower your left forearm parallel to the right shin bone and hold onto the right ankle **(photo # 3-A).**

6. **Option (photo # 3-b):** For a greater twist, reach behind your back with your right hand and reach under your bent right knee with your left hand – striving to clasp hands behind you back **(photo # 3-B).**

<u>Cat 8 / # 4 - Noose Posture (*Pashasana*):</u>

The word *Pasha* relates to a "rope made into a noose." In this posture you will take on the appearance of a noose, as you create a relaxing spinal twist.

Benefits:

In the Noose Posture you will stretch your Achilles tendons, tone and strengthen your spine as well as removing tension from your lower back. This pose is therapeutic for asthma, indigestion, and menstrual discomfort. Stretches and strengthens ankles. This asana also opens chest and shoulders, while improving posture.

Modifications:

Try sitting on a yoga block and choose not to bind in the pose, yet simply wrap your right arm around the outside of your bent knees.

Vinyasa: <u>Hard</u>-Vin # 2-B (Pg 53); <u>Soft</u>- Vin # 5 (Pg 57 - 58)
    Inhale twist away and exhale move into the pose

Cautions: Injury to Knee, Back, Ankle and Neck; plus precautions for Pregnancy.

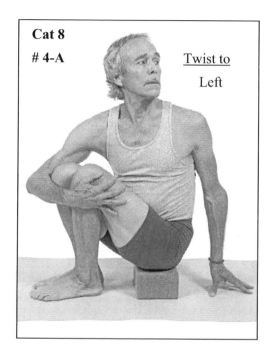

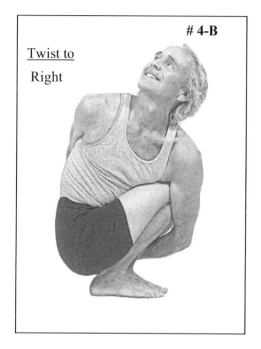

Instructions: <u>Noose Pose – Cat 8 / # 4 (Pg 184 – 185)</u>

1. From Seated Angle Pose **(Pg 87, Photo # 2-A),** bend both knees as you come to a squatting position, with feet flat on the Floor. **Beginner sit on block (photo # 4-A).**

2. Twist your torso to your right side, wrapping your right arm around the knees, with your left hand resting on the floor **(photo # 4-A)**. Less flexible stay here for 5 breaths, or continue on to option 4-B.

3. **Advanced:** Wrap your left arm around both knees and bind with hands reaching behind your back, grabbing right wrist with left hand **(photo # 4-B). Demo is right twist**.

4. Hold this position for five complete breaths on each side, then exhale and relax back to Seated Angle pose, or move through a vinyasa.

Cat 8 / # 5 - The Sage Twist (*Bharadvajasana*):

Bharadvaja was "a wise seer" who is believed to have composed hymns that were later collected in "ancient scriptures" called the *Vedas*, around 1500 BCE. This pose named and dedicated to the Sage *Bharadvaja*, or The Sage Twist.

Benefits:

The Sage Pose stretches the spine, torso, shoulders, and hips. With awareness, this asana can be acceptable and a safe twist for women who are pregnant. This asana improves digestion, regulates metabolism, and aids the organs in detoxification. The Sage Twist also helps to relieve lower back pain, neck pain, and sciatica.

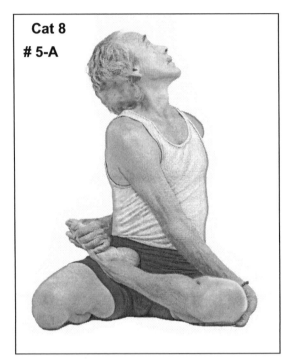

Cat 8
5-A

Cautions:

- Knees injury
- Hip injury
- Back injury
- Neck injury
- Stiff ankles

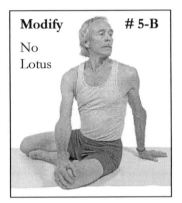

Modify   # 5-B

No Lotus

Modifications:

Try propping your hips up on a blanket or folded yoga mat. This will ease the tension on your back and sensitive knees. If your hips are not open, skip the ½ lotus and just leave your left foot resting against the right inner thigh.

Vinyasa: Hard-Vin # 2-B **(Pg 53); Soft**- Vin # 5 - **(Pg 57 – 58)**

Inhale twist away and Exhale move into the pose.

Instructions: Sage Twist – Cat 8 / # 5 (Pg 185 – 187)

1. Begin seated on the floor with your legs extended in front of you, in Seated Angle pose **(Pg 87, photo # 2-A),** with arms resting at your sides.

2. Bend your right knee, with heel to the outside of your right buttocks; as you bend your left knee, place the bottom of your left foot on your right inner thigh. **Beg**. - Stay here placing your right hand on your left knee and left hand on the floor behind your hips. See **(photo # 5-B, Pg 186)**.

3. **Advanced:** If you have open hips, knees and ankles, place your left foot on top of your right thigh in ½ lotus. Then extend right hand to rest on the outside of your left knee.

4. Then wrap your left arm behind your back, as you try to grasp your left toes with your left hand.

5. Twist your torso to the left as you gaze slightly upward **(photo # 5-A)**. Hold for 5 breaths on each side then return to Seated Angle Pose.

CATEGORY # 9 – ARM BALANCE POSTURES (PG 187 – 206)

Cat 9 / # 1 - Four Limbed Staff (*Charuranga Dandasana*):

In *Sanskrit* language, the word *chatur* which means "four," *anga* meaning "limb," and "danda" means "staff." In this yoga pose, your spine and arms are the main support and will resemble a "rod or staff" supported with 2 hands and 2 feet. The Four Limbed Staff pose.

Benefits:
Strengthens and tones the wrists, arms, abdominal muscles, and lower back. In addition, this pose strengthens the muscles surrounding the spine, which helps to improve posture.

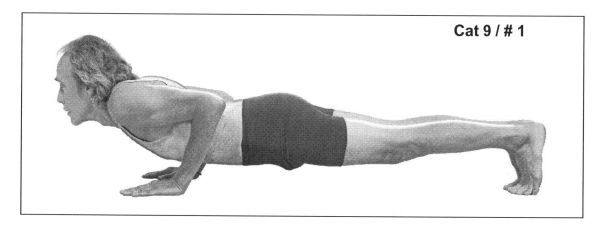

Cat 9 / # 1

Cautions: Injury to Shoulder, Elbow and Ankles; also precautions for Pregnancy.

Modifications:

Place a block or folded blanket up under your thighs, or hips for support - and to create less bend in the wrist, elevate your wrist on a yoga wedge, so that the heel of your palm is higher than your fingers.

Vinyasa:

<u>Enter and exit through any Sun Salutation **(Pg 104 - 111)**, or just Up-dog to Down-dog.</u>

Instructions: <u>**Four Limbed Staff Pose – Cat 9 / # 1 (Pg 187 – 188)**</u>

1. Begin in High Plank (High push-up position) **(Pg 189 - photo # 2)**. Keeping your elbows directly over your wrists, exhale and slowly lower your body to hover a few inches above the floor. Keep your back flat.

2. Be sure to keep your shoulders and abdominals strong, with chest and knees about 3 inches off the floor **(photo # 1).**

3. Sometimes keep elbows to the sides parallel to rib cage, other practice sessions allow elbows to move outward. This creates diversity and results in less injury. Hold for 5 breaths, and then relax on your stomach, or move through a vinyasa.

<u>Cat 9 / # 2 - High Plank Pose (*Kumbhakasana*):</u>

The asana name comes from the Sanskrit words *Kumbhak*, which means "breath retention," and *asana*, which means "pose." Through the yoga tradition in this pose, you would hold your breath for a brief moment before lowering your body down into the low push-up position, *Chaturanga Dandasana* **(photo # 1).** This pose is used often in Sun Salutations and Vinyasa.

Benefits:

This asana tones the core muscles, including the abdomen, chest, and low back. High Plank strengthens the arms, wrists, and shoulders, and also strengthens the muscles surrounding the spine, which improves posture. With regular practice the Plank Pose builds endurance and stamina, while toning the nervous system.

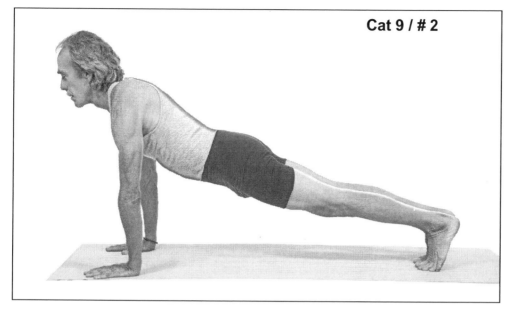

Cat 9 / # 2

Cautions:

- Wrist injury
- Osteoporosis
- Shoulder injury

Modifications:

Try keeping one, or both knees, on the floor for support until you gain more strength. If your wrists get soar, place a yoga wedge under bottom of palms to create less bend in the wrist.

Vinyasa:

Enter and exit through any Sun Salutation, or just use – Up-dog to Down-dog to Plank.

Instructions: <u>High Plank Pose & Side Plank -Cat 9 / # 2 (Pg 188 – 190)</u>

1. Start this asana on your hands and knees, with your wrists directly under your shoulders. Breathe and relax, engage your core and straighten your legs, striving to create one strong line from the top of your head, down to your toes.

2. Spread your fingers wide, and press down through your forearms and hands. Keep your torso and knees straight and strong. Gaze down between your hands and lengthen the back of your neck, then draw your abdominal muscles toward your spine **(photo # 2).**

3. Hold for 5 breaths, then relax on your stomach, or move through a vinyasa.

4. **Options- Side Plank (*Vasisthasana*) (photo # 2-B, C):** *Vasistha* means "most excellent," or "best and richest." Vasistha is the name of several well-known sages in the yoga

tradition. Vasistha is said, also, to be the owner of the fabulous "cow of plenty, *Nandini* "to delight," which grants his every wish and accounts for all his infinite wealth.

5. **Follow the same instructions as above (# 1 – 2),** then place all your weight on your left hand and now turn your torso sideways, to rest on your left hand, keeping hips elevated off the floor and squared to the side, with right hand resting on right hip. Stack your feet, or run feet one in front of the other - **Beginners Stay Here, (photo # 2-B 1).**

6. **Advanced:** Lift your right leg straight upward, perpendicular to the floor and grasp your right big toe with your right 1st and 2nd fingers. Gaze upward at your foot, open your chest and relax for 5 breaths on each side **(photo # 2-B).**

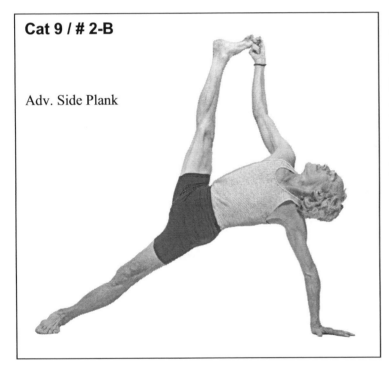

Cat 9 / # 2-B

Adv. Side Plank

As an option – bend your right knee and grasp the knee with your right hand, instead of toes.

If you have a wrist problem, rest on your left bent forearm, instead of your hand.

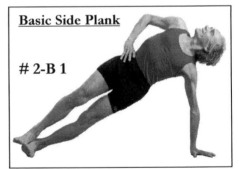

Basic Side Plank

 # 2-B 1

Cat 9 / # 3 - Downward-Facing Dog (*Adho Mukha Svanasana*):

In translation, the word *Adho* means "downward," *mukha* means "face," and *svan* is a "dog." It's named after the way dogs stretch their bodies naturally. Downward Facing Dog is sometimes called "Downward Dog" or just "Down-dog." Downward Facing Dog pose is considered to be in the category of partial arm balances, due to the arm support needed.

Benefits:

This asana energizes and rejuvenates almost the entire body, by deeply stretching your hamstrings, shoulders, calves, arches, hands, and spine while building strength in your arms, shoulders, and legs. Down-dog relieves headaches, insomnia, fatigue, and mild depression. The easy flow of blood to the brain also calms the nervous system, improves memory and relieves stress. Additionally, this asana can improve digestion and relieve back pain.

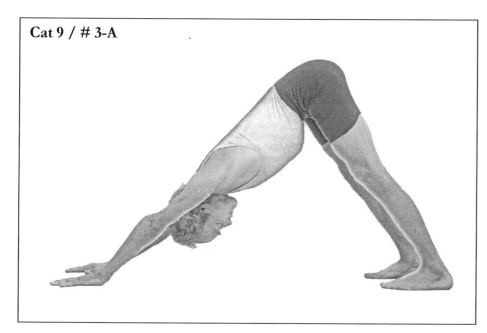

Cat 9 / # 3-A

Cautions:
- Wrist injury
- Shoulder injury
- Eye injury
- Pregnancy
- Blood pressure

Modifications:

Place a yoga wedge under your heels and a yoga block under the top of your head as you bend your knees slightly.

Vinyasa: Enter from any Sun Salutation flow, or just use Up-dog to Down-dog.

Instructions: <u>Downward Facing Dog, and Wild Thing – Cat 9 / # 3 (Pg 190 – 192)</u>

1. Start from a position resting on hands and knees. Align your wrists directly under your shoulders and your knees directly under your hips. Point your fingers facing forward.
2. Now slowly straighten your knees, spread your fingers wide and gaze at feet, as you press the floor away from you lifting through hips, lengthening the entire spine **(photo # 3-A).**
3. Hold for 5 breaths then relax into Child's Pose **(Pg # 94),** or move on to a vinyasa.

Andrea Snyder

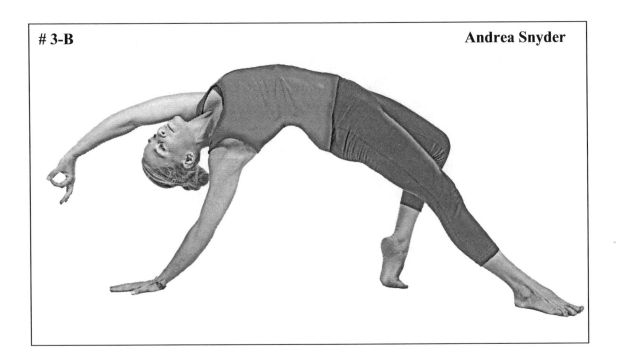

4. **Option: Down-dog Crunches -** Start from Downward Dog Pose **(photo 3-A).** Lift your right leg back and up on the same line with your torso – hold 5 breaths, then exhale and bring your right knee to touch your right elbow; now inhale and return to down-dog - repeat on the opposite side.

5. **Option (# 3-B) – Wild Thing:** Start in Downward Facing Dog **(photo # 3-A).** Lift your left leg up and arch over to the right, placing your left foot on the floor - move further and lift your left hand up. The left foot will touch the floor with knee bent, as you rest on your left toe. Left arm will lift up on the same arch as your back forming a mudra. Hold for 5 breaths on each side. Move back to Downward Facing Dog between each side.

Cat 9 / # 4 - Peacock Pose (*Mayurasana*) / Plus One Arm Peacock:

The word *Mayura* means "peacock" and *asana* means "pose," and in this asana you will take on the beauty and poise of a peacock as it proudly spreads its feathers.

Benefits:

This asana tones up the abdominal portion of the body. It also strengthens the forearms, back, wrists, and elbows. Peacock also teaches balance and coordination.

Modifications:

Place a block, or bolster under your hips and knees, or place your feet onto a block. Another assist is to strap your elbows together so as to keep them from slipping out.

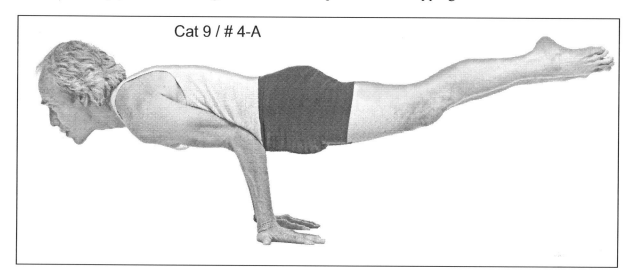

Cat 9 / # 4-A

Cautions:

Injury to Wrist, Elbow and Shoulder: follow precautions in Pregnancy.

Vinyasa:

Use Vin # 4 [(Pg 55) Steps 1-3], then move into Peacock Pose

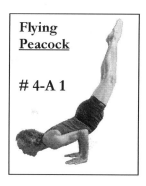

Flying Peacock

4-A 1

Instructions: Peacock Pose – Cat 9 / # 4 (Pg 192 – 194)

1. Start from hands and knees- then begin to twist your hands outward, with fingers facing toward your feet, as you place your elbows up underneath your torso.

2. Now slowly start to straighten your legs, as you put more weight of your torso onto your elbows, forearms, wrists and hands.

3. On an exhalation, lean forward and try to lift your legs and feet up off the floor, balancing parallel to the ground.

4. It is difficult to breathe fully in this position, so make an extra effort to breathe and relax. Hold for 5 breaths **(photo #4-A),** then relax into the Child's Pose, or move to a vinyasa.

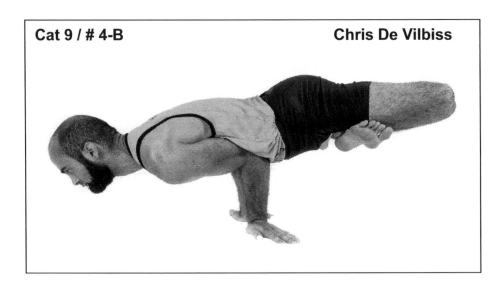

Cat 9 / # 4-B   Chris De Vilbiss

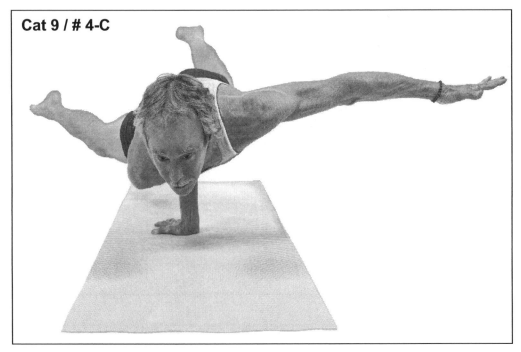

Cat 9 / # 4-C

5. **Option (# 4-B)** Lotus Peacock (*Padma Mayurasana*). Place your legs in Lotus Position before you move into your pose, then place your elbows under your torso and lean forward to balance **(Photo # 5-B).** Hold for 5 Breaths.

6. **Option (# 4-C)** One Arm Peacock: Place right elbow to the center line of your abdominals and your other arm out in front, or off to one side. Now move feet apart and shift your weight forward - try to balance **(photo # 4-C).** Hold for 5 breaths on each side.

Cat 9 / # 5 - Scale Pose (*Tolasana*):

The Sanskrit word *Tola* means a "Pair of Scales" and *asana* means "pose." In this asana you will resemble the old, weigh scale system, like a see-saw, as you balance your body's weight.

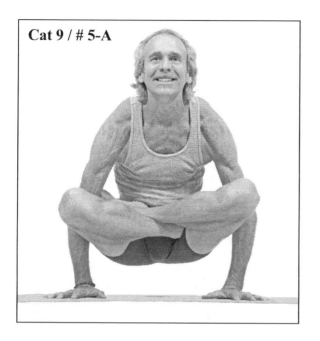

Cat 9 / # 5-A

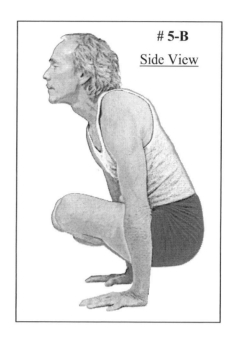

5-B
Side View

Benefits:
Tolasana is an excellent posture for strengthening your stomach, wrists, arms, and shoulders. This posture is a great strengthening exercise and is sometimes used as a training exercise for other arm balancing asana.

Modifications:
Instead of placing your feet in lotus, simply cross your legs and allow your feet to touch the floor, as you push down with your hands. For greater elevation, try placing your hands onto yoga blocks. Or use a yoga wedge under your hands to reduce the backward stretch on the wrist.

Cock Pose - # 5-C – Weave hands through

Your lotus legs and balance on hands, 5 breaths.

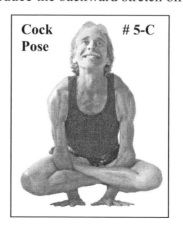

Cock Pose   # 5-C

Vinyasa:

Use **Soft**: Vin # 4 - **(Pg 55)** / Steps 1 -3

or **Hard:** Vin 2-B - **(Pg 53),** then to Scale Pose.

Cautions:

Injury to: Wrist, Shoulder or Elbow. Also, precautions for Pregnancy

Instructions: <u>Scale Pose – Cat 9 / # 5 (Pg 195 – 196)</u>

1. Start this asana from Perfect Posture **(Pg 88, photo # 3),** sitting on the floor in a cross-legged position, then slowly and mindfully place your legs into lotus position.

2. If you cannot do lotus, simply stay in Perfect Posture, then place your hands onto the floor, to the outside of your hips. Now engage your abdominals, as you push down with your hands, trying to lift your torso up off the floor.

3. If you have difficulty lifting your body with your hands, put some blocks under your hands to give yourself some extra lift.

4. While your body is suspended, try lifting your knees up toward your chest and hold this position for five to ten complete breaths, or more **(photo # 5-A / 5-B).**

5. **Cock Pose (*Kukkutasana*):** Weave hands and arms through lotus legs **(photo 5-C).**

6. When finished, lower your hips and knees back to the floor, straighten out your legs and relax into Corpse Posture **(Pg 206),** or move through a vinyasa.

<u>Cat 9 / # 6 - Feather of Peacock (*Pincha Mayurasana*):</u>

The word *Pincha* means "feather," *Mayura* is a "peacock" and *asana* means "pose." When practicing this asana you will resemble the peacock as it lifts its tail into the air, just before spreading its beautiful feathers.

Benefits:

Strengthens abdominals, back, shoulders and arms, at the same time teaches balance and coordination. The expanding of the chest, opens the heart and helps you relax. The legs and buttocks are also strengthened because of the need to keep your body in a straight line.

Cautions: Injury to Back, Shoulder or Neck and high Blood Pressure.

Modifications:

Practice the (Down-dog Pose), only resting on your elbows and forearms, instead of the hands, this will create strength for Feather of Peacock. Try the asana using a wall for support, in front or behind you. Some use a block between the hands to keep elbows from moving outward.

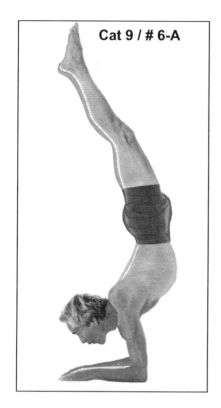

Cat 9 / # 6-A

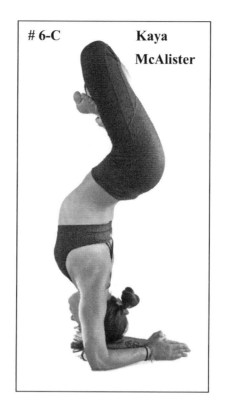

6-C   Kaya McAlister

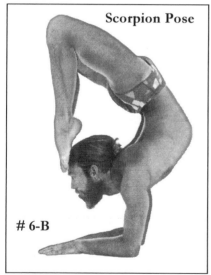

Scorpion Pose

6-B

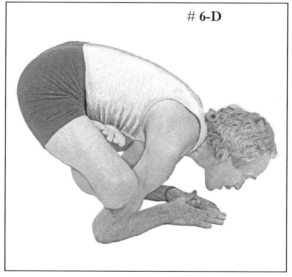

6-D

Vinyasa:

Use **Soft:** Vin # 4 **(Pg 55)** Steps 1 -3

or **Hard:** Vin 2-B **(Pg 53),** then move to Pose.

Instructions: Feather of Peacock – Cat 9 / # 6 (Pg 196 – 198)

1. Start in a position resting on your knees. Then lean forward placing the elbows and forearms flat on the floor with the palms facing down. Your elbows should be placed at least one foot apart, with forearms almost parallel to one another.

2. Now lift your hips upward and extend your head and shoulders forward, as you stay strong in arms. With hands firmly on the floor, keep one knee bent as you prepare to move into the asana.

3. Then either swing one leg up at a time, or press both legs up. Try to maintain your balance and strive to bring the legs up over your head to find your balance. **(photo # 6-A) Feather of Peacock**. Hold for 5 breaths then rest in Child's pose.

4. **Option- Scorpion Pose (photo # 6-B):** From Feather of Peacock, bend your knees and lower the bottoms of feet toward your head **(photo # 6-B)**. Hold 5 breaths

5. **Option- Lotus Feather of Peacock (photo # 6-C):** From Feather of Peacock, try to bend your knees and place feet in lotus **(photo # 6-C)**. Hold 5 Breaths

6. **Option- Duck Pose (photo# 6-D) (*Karandavasana*):** From Scorpion Pose place your legs into full lotus, then lower legs down, to rest knees on your triceps **(photo # 6-D)**. Hold this position for 5 breaths, then press back to Scorpion and relax to Childs Pose.

Cat 9 / # 7 - Crane Pose (*Bakasana*)

The word *Baka* means "crane" In the initial variation of this posture, you resemble a crane wading in a quiet pond with golden sunlight reflecting off the water.

Benefits:

The Crane is great for building your stomach, arm, and shoulder muscles. This posture will also strengthen your wrists, abdominal muscles and improve your balance.

Modifications:

Practice with feet on the ground. Another great modification, is to elevate both of your feet on a yoga block and place a bolster in front of you, if you fall your head will simply rest on the bolster.

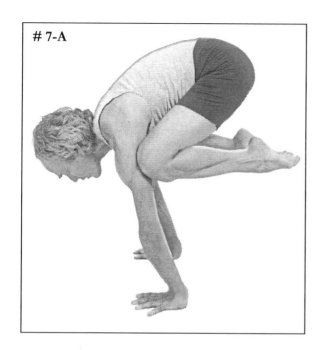

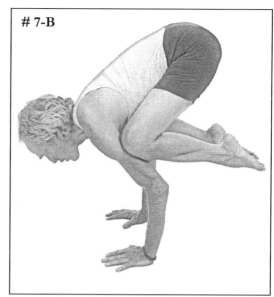

Vinyasa:

Use **Soft** Vin # 4 [(**Pg 55**) Steps 1 -3] or **Hard** Vin 2-B **(Pg 53),** then move to Pose.

Advanced - Can jump in from Down-Dog, or float down from Handstand **(Pg 201)**

Instructions: **Crane Pose – Cat 9 / # 7 (Pg 198 – 200)**

1. Start this posture from Downward Facing Dog **(Pg 190, photo # 3).** Begin by walking your feet a bit closer to your hands, bending your elbows and knees as you gently lower your knees to touch the outside of your elbows.

2. Spread your fingers wide for better support. Keeping your elbows slightly bent, form a ledge to rest your knees upon.

3. Lean your torso forward as you drop your head and shoulders downward, taking some of the weight off your feet and more of your body weight onto your elbows with your knees.

4. Keep pushing gently forward with your toes and try to balance your knees on your elbows, or triceps - as you lift your feet off the floor **(photo # 7-B).**

5. **Advanced students** - straighten the elbows and lift hips upwards – using the abdominals and upper arm strength **(photo # 7-A).**

6. There are many variations to suit different body types, levels of practice and desires. Try to practice a new pose for cross-training and mental flexibility.

7. Try to rotate the variations of the asana at different practice sessions, which will create balance, less chance of injury and greater progress. **(Hold all options for 5 breaths on each side).**

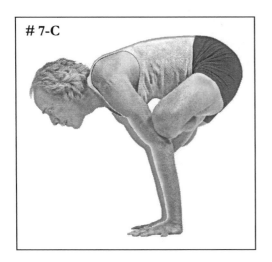

7-C

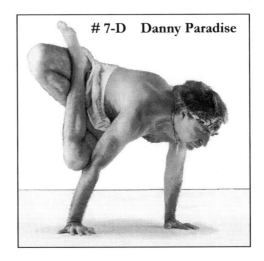

7-D   Danny Paradise

8. **Option- Try Lotus Crane (photo # 7-C):** Place legs in lotus and slowly lift knees to rest above your elbows, or enter from Handstand **(Cat 9 # 8)** and float down to Crane.

9. **Option- Try Side Lotus Crane (photo # 7-D):** From 7-C go to a 3-point headstand and press down to your right side to balance.

10. **Option- Try Side Crane (photo # 7-E):** Go to a 3-point headstand and then press down to your right side, with legs straight and balance for 5 breaths.

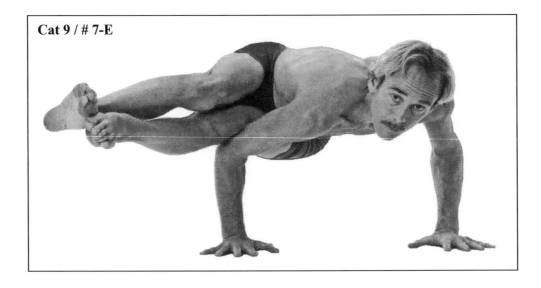

Cat 9 / # 7-E

Cat 9 / # 8 - Handstand Pose (*Adho Mukha Vrkasana*):

The words *Adho Mukha* means "facing downwards" and *Vrksa* means "tree." In this posture, you resemble an upside-down tree with its roots up in the air. This posture is for intermediate or advanced students.

Benefits:

The handstand builds strength and balance as it develops your chest and strengthens your shoulders, arms, and wrist. This posture is also a wonderful way to build your self-confidence.

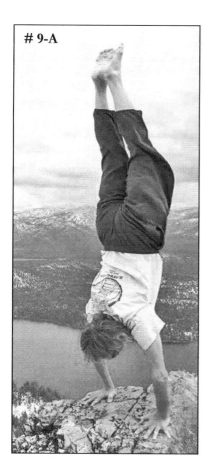

9-A

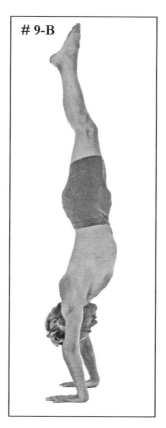

9-B

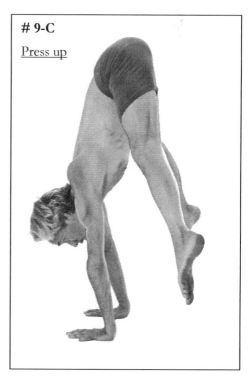

9-C

Press up

Always use caution: do not practice the handstand until your arms can support your weight

Or use a wall with one leg on the floor / or just Down-dog Pose.

Modifications:

Beginner: Practice Downward Facing Dog by itself, or with the heels of your feet at the base of a wall behind you. Then place one leg extended up the wall, with foot flexed, as you place more weight on your hands and arms. **Intermediate:** Another good modification for intermediate level is to kick up to handstand, with a wall behind you for support. It's best to have a spotter to assist you.

Instructions: <u>**Handstand Pose – Cat 9 / # 8 (Pg 201 - 203)**</u>

1. Start from Downward Facing Dog **(Pg 190, photo # 3),** resting on your hands and feet. **Beginners:** Stay here, or position your feet at the base of a wall which is behind you. Stabilize your balance and place one of your feet on the wall about 2- 3 feet off the floor.

2. If comfortable, lift your other foot up onto the wall, keeping arms strong and abdominals engaged. Form a ninety-degree angle with torso, and legs, while keeping feet on the wall.

3. Practice lifting alternate legs up toward the ceiling, one at a time. Hold this position for five complete breaths. When finished, while exhaling, lower your legs back to the ground and relax into Child's Pose.

4. **Intermediate:** If you are stable with your handstand, you can practice on your own by kicking up with the wall behind your back for support.

5. **Advanced:** Try kicking or pressing up, from a standing, forward fold position without the security of the wall **(photo # 9-C).**

6. Strive to drop your head down and look out parallel to the floor, or close your eyes. Keep your spine straight and arms engaged, feel the energy from the Earth and try to relax **(photo 9-A / 9-B).**

7. Hold this posture for five to ten deep breaths, practice two repetitions then exhale, come down slowly and relax into the Child's pose, or move through vinyasa.

Handstand Cautions: Injury to Elbow, Shoulder and Wrist. Also, use precautions for Pregnancy, Eye injury, Glaucoma and high Blood Pressure.

<u>Vinyasa for Handstand see **(Pg 203)**</u>

Handstand Vinyasa: Use **Soft** Vin # 4 & # 5 **(Pg 55 – 57),** or **Hard** Vin 2-B **(Pg 53),** then move into the pose. **Or** you can move through a Sun Salutation, then enter into handstand. **Adv:** can press up to pose - Step # 5 **(Pg 202).**

Cat 9 / # 10 - Flying Insect (*Tittibhasana*):

The word *Tittibha* refers to a "Flying Insect," and in this yoga posture you will take on the characteristics and energy of a flying insect, as you spread your wings and fly.

Benefits:

Insect is a good leg stretch along with strengthening arms, shoulders, abdominals and wrists. The Flying Insect also teaches balance, coordination and the concept of softness is strength.

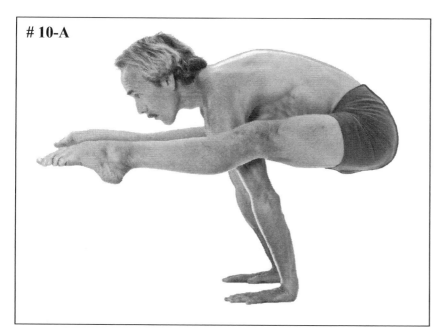

10-A

Cautions:

- Wrist injury
- Elbow injury
- Shoulder injury
- Pregnancy

Modifications:

Practice the Crane Pose on **(Pg 199, photo # 7-A, 7-B),** as an option. Another modification is to sit upon a few blocks to elevate your hips up off the floor, then place your hands onto the floor and lean forward, as you try to lift your buttocks up off the blocks. Students with shorter arms can place blocks under your hands.

Vinyasa:

Easy: Vin # 4 – **(Pg 55, 56)** Steps 1 – 3; **Hard:** Jump in from Down-dog, or float down from Handstand. **Adv:** Exit using Flying Vinyasa **(Pg 55, photo # 3)** to Handstand, or to 4-Limbed Staff.

Instructions: <u>Flying Insect – Cat 9 / # 10 (Pg 203 – 204)</u>

1. Start from a standing forward fold, with a wide stance, placing your hands on the floor between your feet and slightly behind the heels. Then, as you bend your knees, lowering your hips down toward the floor, as you rest your hamstrings on your elbows.

2. Be strong through your hands and arms, as you engage your abdominals and find your balance. Hold this position for five complete breaths **(photo #10-A).** When you are finished lower your torso mindfully back to the floor and relax into Child's Pose, or move though a vinyasa.

3. **Advanced Students** - press down into Flying Insect from Handstand Pose, or press up from Tortoise Pose.

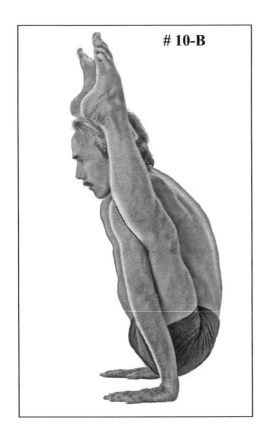

10-B

4. **<u>Option</u>– Vertical Flying Insect (photo 10-B).** From (Photo # 10-A), lower your hips toward the floor as you lift your feet upward – trying not to touch the floor **(photo # 10-B).** Gaze forward and Hold for 5 breaths.

5. **<u>Advanced</u>**- Exit by jumping back into Four-Limbed Staff Pose, or press up to handstand, then float down to Four Limbed Staff.

Cat 9 / Photo # 11 - Crocodile Pose (*Nakarasana*) :

The word *Nakarasana* means "Crocodile" and in this pose you will take on the full energy and essence of a powerful crocodile lunging quickly forward.

As legend has it, some beautiful ladies were dancing sensuously in front of a sage to win his attention – yet he did not like it, and turned them into crocodiles – destined to live their life in the lake as reptiles. People were afraid to sun bath by the lake for fear of being eaten, so Arjuna decided to rid the lake of the crocks and when he grabbed the crocks and wrestled them to the land - they immediately turned back into beautiful ladies.

Even though this asana may seem crusty and rough on the outside, bring it onto the shores of your mind and try to embrace its true inner beauty. ☺

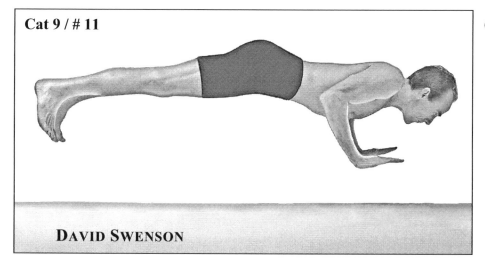

Cat 9 / # 11

DAVID SWENSON

Cautions:

- Wrist injury
- Shoulder injury
- Elbow injury
- Pregnancy

Benefits:

This pose will strengthen wrists, arms, chest and back, while teaching balance and technique. This pose also builds self-confidence and rhythm.

Modifications:

Try Four limbed staff and do half way push-ups quickly, this will build the strength. Another modification is to keep one foot on the floor when you try to jump upward.

Vinyasa: Inhale to Upward Dog, then exhale to Down Dog, then move into the Low Plank.

Instructions: <u>Crocodile Pose – Cat 9 / # 11 (Pg 205 – 206)</u>

1. Start in Four Limbed Staff Pose **(Pg 187, photo # 1),** next using the concept of doing a quick push-up push, hop or lunge forward and backward, using the momentum of your hips, and power of our hands, feet and abdominals.

2. Be careful not to injure your wrist, as you lunge 3 – 4 times forward and back again **(photo # 11).** Inhale when you lunge and exhale when you land.

3. When you finish, inhale and take a vinyasa to Up Dog and then exhale and back to Down Dog; rest in Child's Pose for a few breaths, or go on to your next asana.

CATEGORY # 10 DEEP RELAXATION (PG 206 – 210)

<u>Category 10 / # 1 - Corpse Pose (*Savasana*):</u>

The Sanskrit name, *Savasana*, comes from two words: *Sava* meaning "corpse," and *asana* meaning "pose." The other name is known as Sponge Pose; because you will be resting on your back soaking up healing energy from the mother earth. This is the final pose of almost every yoga asana class. The Corpse Pose: dedicated to deep relaxation and restoration of body, mind and spirit.

The Corpse Pose reflects a depth of release that goes beyond just simple relaxation.

This relaxation pose takes your body and mind to a place where you can completely let go, with the feeling of being refreshed, revitalized and reborn. Make sure you end every yoga practice with the **Corpse Posture (Pg 207)** and **Deep Relaxation Technique on (page 208)**.

On **(page 207 # 10)** you will find an example of the Corpse Pose.

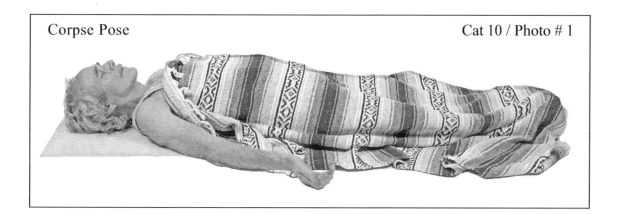

Corpse Pose   Cat 10 / Photo # 1

Very often, many yoga students find it difficult to lie completely still, while being both fully aware and unattached from any distractions. Mastering this amazing technique of deep relaxation can take time, practice and patience, and yet the rewards are truly a priceless gift.

Unlike the active, moving, and sometimes physically demanding poses, the Corpse Pose requires a conscious decision from you to release the mental chatter and surrender fully into a state of total and complete blissful relaxation.

All yoga asana traditions and yoga teachers should regard *savasana* as the single most important pose of your whole asana practice. For many reasons, yet mostly, it allows your body time to process the information and benefits received from the yoga asana practice and breathing exercises. This wonderful technique, offers more than just the physical aspects, this technique enhances and renews the, mind, and spirit, which will touch every aspect of your daily life in a very positive way.

Benefits:

Lowers blood pressure, decreases heart rate, and fosters slower and deeper breathing. This practice also decreases muscle tension while gaining mental clarity and inner peace, as you release stress and mental tension. The practice of yoga deep relaxation has been known to increase self-confidence, and promote healing in the body, while embracing positive thinking.

Cautions:

Corpse pose is appropriate for almost all yoga students, unless you are pregnant; in which case you should keep your head and chest raised in the pose by resting on your side, and on a bolster or a few pillows.

Props You Might Need:

You can practice Corpse Pose with no props at all and have a most wonderful experience; however, many students choose to enjoy the use of yoga props and a controlled environment to make an easier transition into a state of bliss. **If you choose to use props then it is best to have these things in order and readily available, beforehand.**

    (a) **Props** - Bolster, pillows, blankets, and an eye pillow are all quite useful.

    (b) **Environment** – Temperature, music, fresh air and aroma therapy. I personally do not burn incense, because this will place burned ash into the air, and in essence, you are polluting the air; in order to mask less appealing smells, instead try essential oils, or fresh flowers.

The body temperature will decrease in deep relaxation, and so you may want to use a blanket and a pair of socks before settling into the practice. Try placing a bolster, or folded blanket underneath your knees, which takes weight off of your pelvis, and low back. The use of an eye pillow can also add to a more restful deep relaxation exercise.

Cat 10 / # 2 - Deep Relaxation Technique   (Page # 208 – 210)

Instructions:

1. Lie on your back with your legs straight, feet resting apart and arms at your sides, with palms facing upward. Rest your hands about six inches away from your body and allow your feet to drop open, as your shoulders melt into the floor. Then close your eyes, relax your mind and release your thoughts.
2. Let your breathing occur naturally, light and smooth, and with relaxed awareness, as you allow your body to surrender to the earth.
3. Now lift your right leg about 12 inches from the floor, tense every muscle in your leg for a few seconds then exhale, relax, and gently lower your leg to the floor. Repeat this step with your left leg.

4. Then tighten the muscles in your buttocks for a few seconds, exhale and relax, allowing your gluteus muscles to "melt" into the floor.

5. Now arch your back, pressing down with your elbows and shoulders as you expand your chest toward the ceiling, hold this position for a few seconds, and then exhale, relax and lower your back to rest on the floor.

6. Next you will press your lower back into the floor by tightening your buttocks and stomach muscles, as you press against the floor, hold this position for a few seconds, and then exhale and relax completely.

7. Then continue as you lift your right arm about one foot off the floor, tensing all the muscles, hold this position for a few seconds, and then exhale, relax, and lower your arm to the floor. Repeat this step using your left arm.

8. Now roll your head very slowly to the right, and then back to the left, then return your head to the center, then exhale and relax.

9. As you continue, fill your mouth with air, blowing your cheeks out like balloons hold for a couple of seconds, and then exhale, relax and release the air, as you gently stretch all your facial muscles, and then relax them.

10. **Mental Deep Relaxation**: Making sure your eyes are closed, take five slow, deep breaths and clear your mind.

11. The next phase is to mentally go back over your whole body once again (only this time using only your mind to "relax" starting from the toes and working slowly to the crown of your head, visualize each part of your body, one by one, as you mentally allow each muscle, bone, tendon and organ to relax.

12. This whole technique is greatly enhanced if you visualize drawing energy into your body on inhalations and then releasing stress and tensions on exhalations.

13. Turn your focus internally, visualize your heart, then exhale and mentally ask your heart to relax. Then visualize your brain, as you exhale again to calm and relax your brain by releasing your thoughts.

14. Clear your mind of all but the most pleasant and positive thoughts and visualize a beautiful place in nature and imagine yourself in this scene of beauty. Remain in this state of mind for five to ten minutes.

15. **Coming Back**: When finished, slowly invite some movement back into your toes, then relax for a moment and now slowly invite some movement back into your fingers.

16. Then stretch your arms over your head on an inhalation and as you exhale, roll over onto your right side, with your arms and legs slightly bent. Rest on your right side as you remain in this position for a few relaxing breaths.

17. When you are finished, gradually return to a seated position and try to preserve the positive, uplifting energy and thoughts that you created, carrying this with you throughout the rest of your day.

End Deep Relaxation Exercise

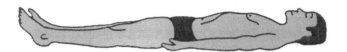

Be The Light

If the desert would give back …
This sand, like a mother's touch of warmth
Yet, cactus just dreams of a watery life
And ask why – as the night whispers

Tomorrow needs our love, our kindness …
And genuine integrity – this flower slow dances
Like a homeless thought, lost between time
Ego fishes for answers but finds no truth

The taste of yesterday's richness
Touched stray mountains – where sunbeams seek peace
It is not enough – to be the love of the wind
We must find the heart in preservation and be the light …

------ *Doug Swenson*

My poem was first featured in
"Poetry of Yoga" / By Hawah"

CHAPTER 6

Practicing Beginner Level Yoga Routines

True enlightenment is found
Within realizing you will always be a student

When you first start practicing Sadhana Vinyasa Yoga, you should not expect to master the whole system in one session. Be patient with yourself. Even if you plan on becoming a yoga teacher, always consider yourself a student for life. In the beginning you may have times when you feel awkward, clumsy, humbled, and even frustrated. However, you will also have many moments where you feel comfortable, at peace; relaxed, and even euphoric, feeling that yoga has become your very best friend.

Remember to enjoy the journey, be in the moment and try to look forward to your practice, as a vacation, not as work. The object **is not** to achieve the most advanced posture, it is to connect with the natural flow of energy, feel good about your-self and develop inner peace. In the beginning it is a good idea to rest between your postures, whenever you feel it is necessary. In time you will create a continuous flow of practice.

HINTS AND SUGGESTIONS FOR BEGINNERS

1. When Seated, if your hips are tight and your leg muscles are not flexible, try placing a small pillow under your hips and if necessary, under your knees as well.

2. Strive to create good posture with awareness in all asana, remember to take your time - relax and allow the soothing touch of yoga energy to become you.

3. Value the exhalation as being just as important as inhalation and make the effort to completely empty your lungs before each inhalation.

4. Draw energy into your body on inhalations and release stress and tension on exhalations.

5. Yoga is about awareness - leave your ego at the door and invite gratitude to join you.

Yoga Beyond the Mat — After your yoga asana practice, try to stay calm and if possible, take a short walk in nature — to move the prana and enjoy the wonderful results of awareness.

Kindness and Karma Yoga — As a beginner, try to strive to be an example of kindness and selfless action; this will help you and others.

Beginner Short Routine: (40 – 50 minute practice)

Practice the following routine by completing each of the exercises and postures listed. Pay attention to the durations for each posture, and strive to hold each pose for the duration given.

Seated Postures and Yoga Breathing: (10 complete breaths)

Yoga Warm-Ups: *(You can choose more or different warm-ups)*

Alternate the Cat Stretch during your first session, and the Sun Salutation at your next session.

Standing Postures

Alternate Triangle Pose at one practice session and the Twisted Triangle at the next.

Inversions and Counter Stretches

Leg Stretches

Remember to be mindful of your breathing, inhale drawing energy into your body and exhale releasing stress and tension as you move slightly deeper into your asana. Use your breathing to assist in all aspects of practice.

Back Bends

Spinal Twist

Deep Relaxation

Beginner Long Routine: (1 hour to 1:30 minute practice)

Practice the following routine by completing each of the exercises and postures listed. Pay attention to the durations for each posture, and strive to hold each pose for the duration given. If you find you do not have enough time to complete this routine in your allotted amount of time, simply skip ahead to the relaxation exercise and then finish the last half of your practice the next session.

Seated Postures and Yoga Breathing

Yoga Warm-up Exercises: *(You can choose more or different warm-ups)*

Standing Postures

Perform all three of the postures listed, in order of sequence.

Inversions and Counter Stretches

Perform all three of the postures listed, in order of sequence.

Leg Stretches

Perform all three of the postures listed, in order of sequence.

Back Bend Postures

Perform all three of the postures listed, in order of sequence.

Spinal Twisting Postures

Breathing and Pranayama

Deep Relaxation (5 – 20 minutes)

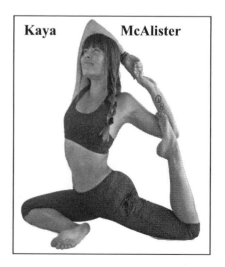

Kaya   McAlister

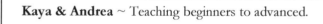

Kaya & Andrea ~ Teaching beginners to advanced.

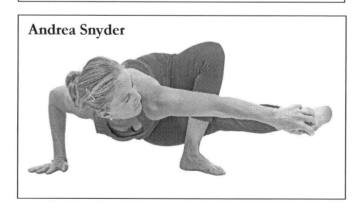

Andrea Snyder

CHAPTER 7

Practicing Intermediate Level Yoga Routines

One brief moment of practice
Is worth more, than a millennium of thought

Intermediate students have acquired some degree of self-confidence and have tasted many of yoga's physical benefits. This background will work to your advantage as you incorporate the lessons of Sadhana Vinyasa Yoga into your yoga practice. Intermediate students should feel free to practice any of the beginner level routines as an alternative to the routines listed in this section. Just as with a beginner practice, don't be intimidated by thumbing ahead to the more extreme postures. There is no evidence to support the notion that those practicing advanced level postures are any more spiritual, wise, or enlightened than those at the beginner, or intermediate level.

It is much more important to have a comfortable, quality practice than to push yourself beyond your current limits and not enjoy the routine. "The path to enlightenment is the middle line."

HINTS AND SUGGESTIONS FOR INTERMEDIATE STUDENTS

1. If your hips are tight and your leg muscles not flexible, try placing a small pillow under your hips and if necessary, under your knees as well. On occasion, try yoga in a hot room, to help with hip flexibility and tight muscles.

2. Strive to create good posture with your shoulders back and with a straight spine. Take your time: relax and enjoy the soothing touch of energy.

3. Try to lengthen your breath and remember that inhalation is just as important as exhalation, so make the effort to completely empty your lungs before each inhalation.

4. Draw energy into your body on inhalations and release stress and tension on exhalations.

5. Review (**Pg 39 – 40)** for complete details on yoga breathing, you will find the seated posture's variations and instructions listed in Chapter 3.

Intermediate Short Routine: (45 to 60 minutes)

Seated Postures and Yoga Breathing:

Perfect Posture or Lotus Posture……………………………………………………………………88, 89

Basic Yoga Breathing (10 complete breaths)…………………………………………..40, 41, 259

Yoga Warm-ups: (*You can choose more or different warm-ups*) Pg 76 - 84

Perform each of the following postures in the order they are listed.

Neck rolls and Shoulder rolls………………………………………………………………...77, 78

Cat Stretch (Two Repetitions)...…………………………………………………………...105, 106

Sun Salutation – Soothing Touch Level #1 (Two Repetitions)…………………...………..107 - 109

Standing Postures:

Perform each of the following postures in the order they are listed.

Revolved Extended Triangle……………………………………………………...………………119

Warrior I…………………………………………………………………………………….129, 130

Inversions and Counter Stretches:

In the intermediate practice, you will find both Headstand and Shoulder Stand postures; try to keep your spine straight drawing one line, which creates a stronger pose.

Leg Stretches:

Perform each of the following postures in the order they are listed.

Back Bends:

Perform each of the following postures in the order they are listed.

Spinal Twist:

Arm Balance:

Breathing and Pranayama

Deep Relaxation:

Always take the time for a quality deep relaxation. Some students find it helpful to use an eye pillow and light, background music.

Intermediate Long Routine (1 hour to 1:30 minute practice)

If you find you do not have enough time to complete this routine, simply take relaxation and finish the last half of your practice the next session.

<u>(Intermediate Long Routine / Begins Here (1 hr – 1:30 Practice)</u>

Sitting and Breathing:

Perfect Posture or Lotus ……………………………………………………………89

Basic Yoga Breathing (10 breaths)………………………………………40, 41, 259

Yoga Warm-up Exercises: *(You can choose more or different warm-ups)*

Please complete each of the following postures in the order as listed.

Neck rolls and Shoulder rolls……………………………………………………77, 78

Cat Stretch (Two Repetitions)…………………………………………………104, 107

Chi Stretch…………………………………………………………………………80

Sun Salutation – Soothing Touch (Four Repetitions)………………………107 - 109

Sun Salutation – Power Zone (Two Repetitions)…………………………110, 111

Standing Postures:

Please complete each of the following postures in the order as listed.

Triangle Pose……………………………………………………………………117

Revolved Triangle Pose………………………………………………………119

Side Angle Pose………………………………………………………………120

Expanded Foot Pose……………………………………………………………123

Warrior I …………………………………………………………………129, 130

Inversions and Counter Stretches:

Please complete each of the following postures in the order as listed.

Headstand………………………………………………………………………140

Fish ……………………………………………………………………………146

Shoulder Stand…………………………………………………………………142

Bridge…………………………………………………………………………144

Leg Stretches:

Staff and Forward bend sitting…………………………………………………100

Back Bend Postures:

Please complete each of the following postures in the order as listed.

Spinal Twisting Postures:

Please complete each of the following postures in the order as listed.

Arm Balance Postures:

Please complete each of the following postures in the order as listed.

Breathing and Pranayama:

Deep Relaxation:

Some students find it helpful to use an eye pillow and light background music.

CHAPTER 8

Practicing Advanced Level Yoga Routines

Seek yoga to soften the jagged stone
And touch the thoughts
That stand alone

Advanced students should strive not only to master the physical skills, but to achieve a spiritual quality within their practice. Make an effort to maintain a full body-mind connection, even during the most difficult routines. Keep peace and compassion in your heart, be non-competitive, and always take time to help the newcomer. Remember you were once a beginner as well.

Pick one teacher as your base, yet study from several different teachers in the larger spectrum of things. No one teacher has all the answers, no matter what they tell you. Even if your teacher is highly recommended, famous and of guru status, if they claim their system is the best ever and encourage you to never seek other instruction, then they have failed at their own yoga practice.

Yoga Beyond the Mat — After your yoga asana practice, try to stay calm, and if possible, take a short walk in nature – to move the prana and enjoy the wonderful results of awareness.

Kindness and Karma Yoga — As an advanced student, you should know and strive to be an example of kindness and selfless action, this will help you *and* others. Go out of our way to be the light in darkness, learn to see the world "through the eyes of another", striving for deeper awareness and communication.

Using Your Yoga Energy — The energy you have created in yoga, can be used in your everyday life with wonderful results, yoga improves all situations and moments. Practice a yogic state of mind with all the following topics and more: at work, with family and relationships, recreation and with hobbies, or special interest. As an advanced student you will find yoga is starting to touch your soul in a positive way. Your mind will be more focused and you will feel almost anything is possible. This mind focus will branch out into your daily life and assist you in every aspect of your existence.

Diet and Nutrition:

As an advanced student, if you are not yet a vegetarian, or vegan you should now make the change, educate yourself and be an inspiration for others. Also try to shun junk food, bad habits and less healthy cuisine.

Advanced Short Routine: (60 – 70 Minutes) *(Less time / practice only ½)*

Sitting and Breathing:

Practice one of the following seated positions best suited for your present condition, and sit quietly, with good posture, for 15 complete breaths. Let your breathing become smooth and fine, as you strive to expand your lungs with slow, deep inhalations and exhalations. As an advanced student, you should try to feel the energy moving through your body and be attentive on embracing a spiritual element. For variety and well-balanced practice, choose a different posture each time you practice.

Seated Postures and Yoga Breathing:

Perfect Posture or Lotus Posture…………………………………..……………...88, 89
Basic Yoga Breathing (10 Complete Breaths)…………………………………....40, 41, 259

Yoga Warm-Ups: *(You can choose more or different warm-ups)*

Standing Postures:

Inversions and Counter Stretches:

Advanced students should be attentive to a smooth entrance and exit with these inversions.

Leg Stretches:

As an Advanced student, you can move deeper into your stretch as you feel the lines of energy opening. Remember to breathe as you are stretching: exhale to release stress and tension, as you move slightly deeper into your stretch; inhale, embracing energy, as you back off from the stretch slightly.

Back Bends:

Spinal Twist:

Arm Balance:

Deep Relaxation:

Advanced Long Routine (1:30 hour to 2 hour practice):

In order to retain the full potential of energy flow, follow this routine from start to finish in the order laid out. Once a month, go back and hold postures for twice the suggest amount of time, in each given routine. If you find you do not have enough time to complete this routine, in your allotted amount of time, simply take relaxation and finish the last half of your practice the next session. An advanced student should be able to connect every posture together with suggested vinyasa from the posture instructions in (Chapter 5).

Sitting and Breathing:

Yoga Warm-up Exercises:

Please follow the order as laid out in this routine below; the postures are listed in order of sequence. Advanced students can cross train with all other warm-ups.

Standing Postures:

In the standing postures, strive to move with your breath and visualize where you are and where you want to go.

Inversions and Counter Stretches:

Complete all of the postures in this section in the order they appear.

Leg Stretches:

Complete all of the postures in this section in the order they appear.

Back Bend Postures:

Complete all of the postures in this section in the order they appear.

Spinal Twisting Seated Postures:

Arm Balance Postures:

Complete all of the postures in this section in the order they appear.

Breathing and Pranayama:

Deep Relaxation (10 – 20 minutes):

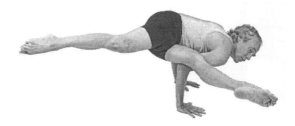

CHAPTER 9

Honoring Yoga Teachers
As Many Hearts Beat as One

In this chapter, I ask every student and teacher alike, to give honor and respect for all the various styles and lineages of yoga practice. Teachers are always giving, so please join me now in celebrating and honoring these wonderful teachers - as the music of their practice, inspires birth of a sacred and beautiful symphony.

Yoga is an art and a mindful discipline, which ultimately enhances every aspect of life, and, it is one that assists to elevate consciousness in all who practice. And yet, most of all, yoga is self-expression, as we find the freedom in what makes us unique. Let us all retain our individuality; and yet, learn to see the world through another's eyes, to create a song of serenity. If you truly listen, you can hear the music, and feel the pulse as many hearts beat as one – in harmony.

I honor the place within your heart where peace prevails. I honor your sacred message as an individual. Most of all, I celebrate your effort and practice as we become one in light, bathing in the melody of peace.

Blessing and Love, Doug Swenson

Seane Corn

 # 9-A

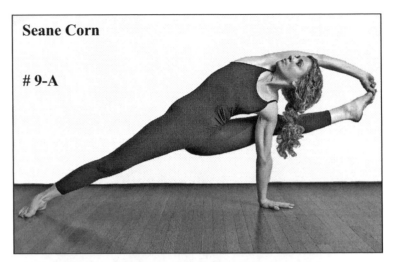

 # 9-B   **Mark Stroud**

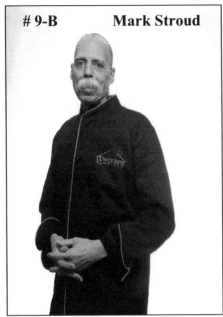

Dharma Mittra

 # 9-C

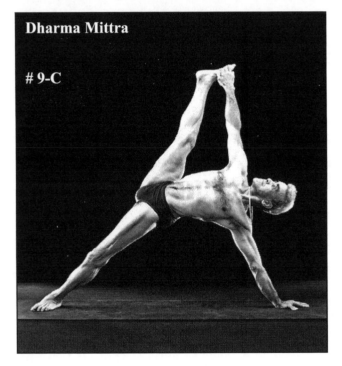

Kaya McAlister

 # 9-E

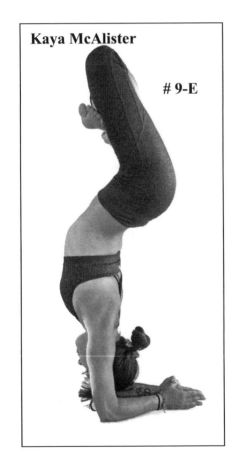

 # 9-D   **Andrea Snyder**

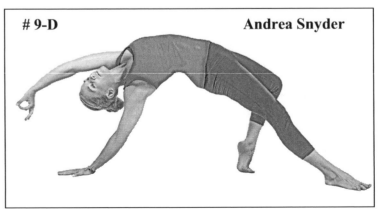

David Swenson # 9-F

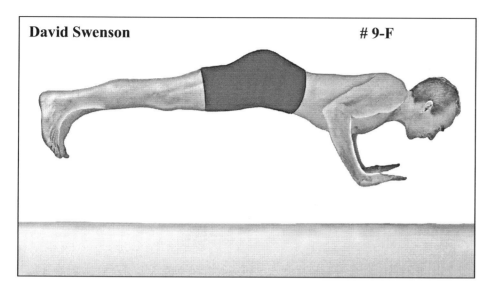

9-F1 David

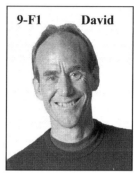

9-I Anna Ferguson

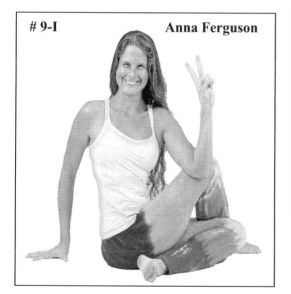

Chris De Vilbiss # 9-H

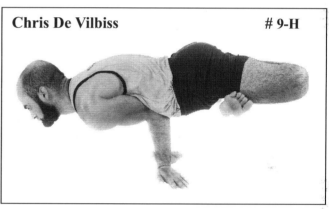

Mayra Cadengo # 9-Z6

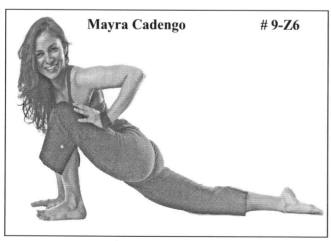

9-G Alex Keller

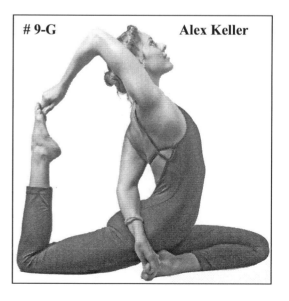

Sara Turk # 9-J

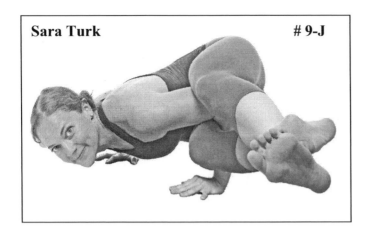

Jonny Kest # 9-K

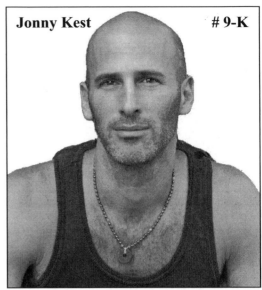

9-L **Sharron Gannon & David Life**

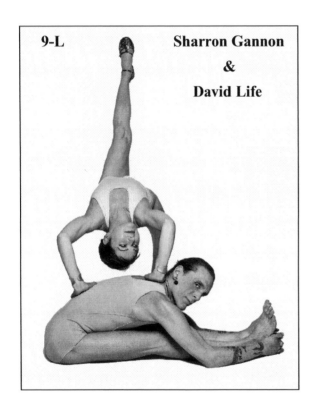

Danny Paradise

9-M

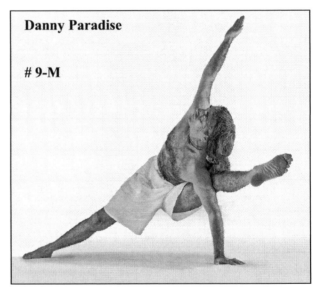

David # 9-N

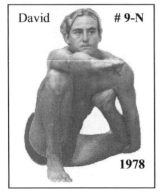

1978

Doug

9-Nn

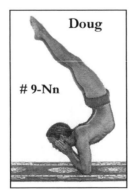

Svetlana Panina # 9-N-1

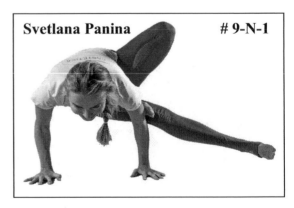

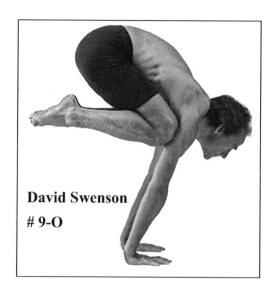

David Swenson
 # 9-O

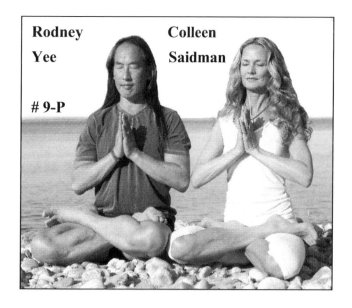

Rodney Yee   **Colleen Saidman**

 # 9-P

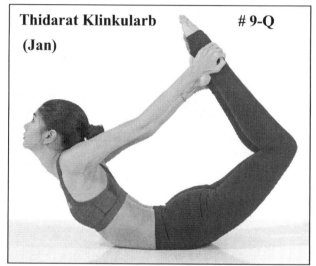

Thidarat Klinkularb   **# 9-Q**
(Jan)

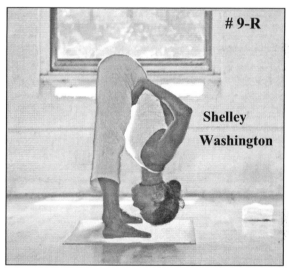

 # 9-R

Shelley Washington

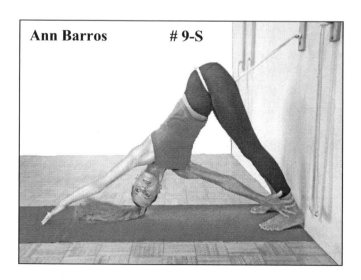

Ann Barros   **# 9-S**

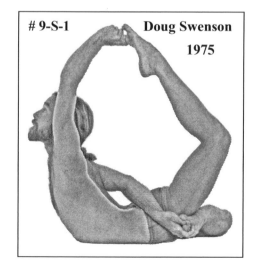

 # 9-S-1   **Doug Swenson 1975**

Tao Porchon   **# 9-T**

Lynch   **Doug**

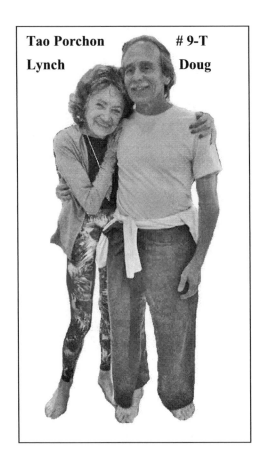

Svetlana Panina   **# 9-U**

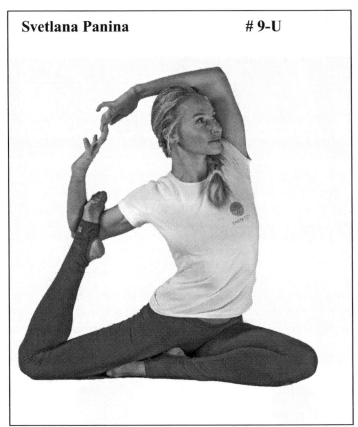

Tao

Porchon

Lynch

 # 9-V

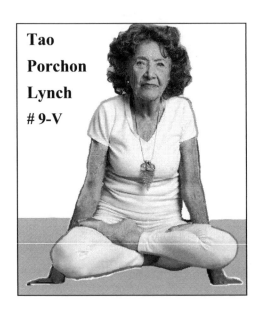

Thidarat Klinkularb   **# 9-W**

(Jan)

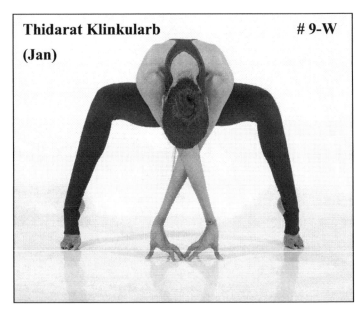

Paul & Suzie Grilley # 9-X

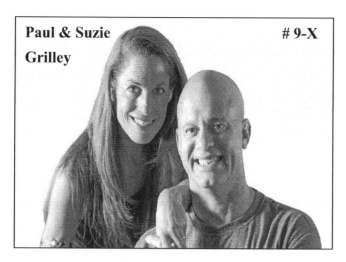

9-Y **Almendra Garcia**

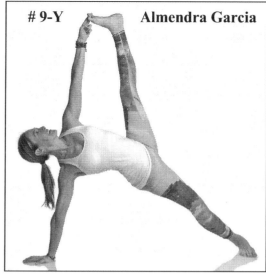

Sara Turk

9-Z

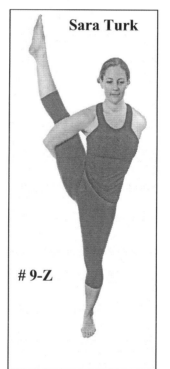

Joy & Ricardo # 9-Z1

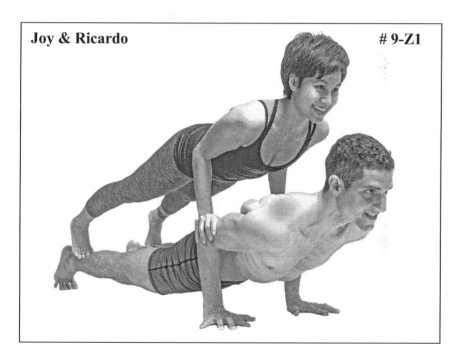

Andrea Snyder

9 –Z

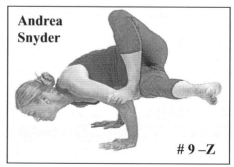

Vi

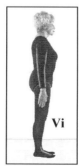

Doug Swenson # 9-Z-1A

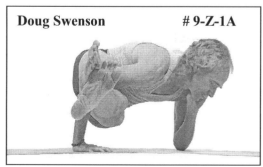

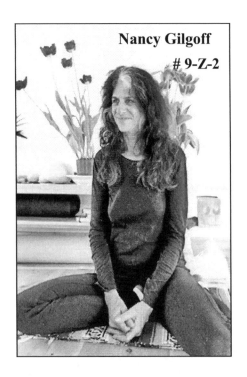

Nancy Gilgoff
 # 9-Z-2

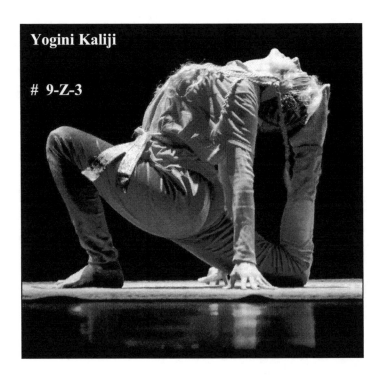

Yogini Kaliji
 # 9-Z-3

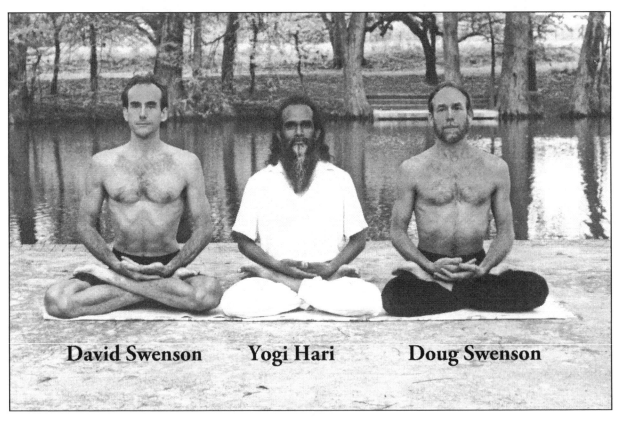

David Swenson **Yogi Hari** **Doug Swenson**

(Photo # 9-Z4)

Shelley Washington # 9-Z-5

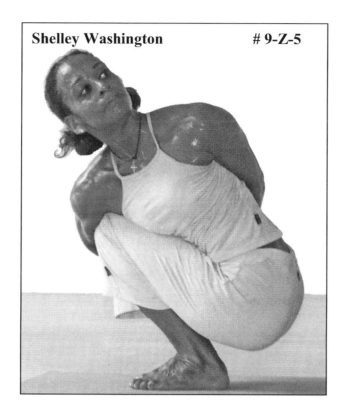

Shelley and David
 # 9 Z- 5A

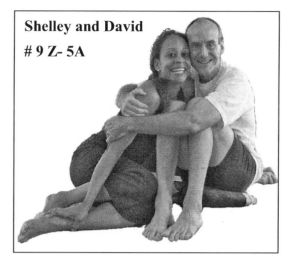

Almendra Garcia

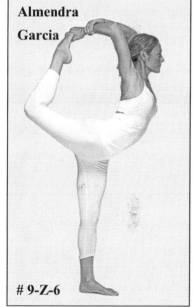

9-Z-6

Mark & Anna
(World Peace Yoga) # 9-Z-7

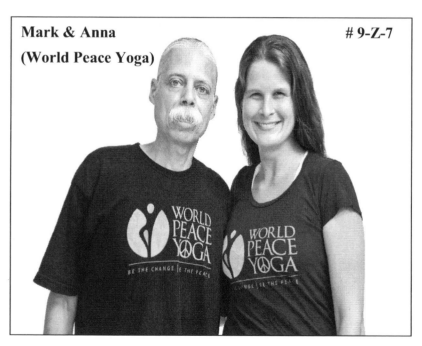

David **Doug**

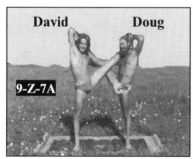

9-Z-7A

Alex Keller - (Alex Keller Yoga) Dayton, Ohio / **(9-G)**

RYT 500, is dedicated to Yoga, Fitness, and everything which Brings Peace, Contentment and Happiness, to life. Teaches: Stand Up Paddle Board Yoga, Spinning, TRX, Kayaking, Water Aerobics, Pilates and Yoga, incorporating all these modalities as a personal trainer.

Contact: Alexkelleryoga@gmail.com / Website: www.Alexkelleryoga.com

Almendra Garcia – (Ashtanga and Hatha Yoga) – Tampico, MX / **(9-Y)**

Founder of Sthira Yoga Center, she began her training in Ashtanga and over time she also studied Hatha, Vinyasa Yoga, Sadhana Vinyasa Yoga, Kundalini and Pilates, which have enriched her teachings. Almendra integrates the aspects of healthy eating into her teaching.

Contact: almendra@sthirayoga.com.mx / www.almendrayoga.com

Andrea C Snyder - (Power, Vinyasa, Bikram, Ashtanga) - Lake Tahoe **(9-D)**

Teaches in South Lake Tahoe CA and Stateline NV, practicing for 20 years - teaching mostly Power, Vinyasa, Bikram, and Ashtanga yoga, with all levels and many formats, keeping an open mind.

Contact: (775) 378-8377 / Yogaphoenix31@gmail.com

Ann Barros - (Iyengar Yoga) - Santa Cruz, CA **(9-S)**

Highest quality certified Iyengar Instructor since 1980, leading Yoga In Bali retreats since 1986.

Contact: abarros@pacbell.net / www.baliyoga.com

Anna Ferguson – (World Peace Yoga) - Cincinatti, OH **(9-I, 9-Z7)**

Director of World Peace Yoga Personal Spiritual Growth and Yoga Teacher Training programs. I have studied with many great teachers to include; Doug Swenson, Julie Kirkpatrick, David Life, Sharon Gannon, and Will Tuttle, PhD.

Contact: yoga@worldpeaceyoga.com / www.worldpeaceyoga.com

Christopher De Vilbiss – (Ashtanga, Sadhana Yoga Chi, Acro) – Gainesville, FL **(9-H)**

A wrestler, Chris found yoga in 2007, practices mostly Ashtanga Yoga, Sadhana Yoga Chi, AcroYoga, and Meditation. He believes that every day his awareness increases and Chris applies this new awareness toward all his physical and mental aspects of life.

Contact: yogiChris@9thlimb.com / www.9thlimb.com

Danny Paradise - (Ashtanga Yoga and Shamanism) - Hawaii **(9-M, Pg 200, Pg 288)**

Practicing Ashtanga Yoga since 1976, in addition to studying Karate, Kung Fu and Tai Chi over the years. Danny's first Yoga teachers were David Williams and Nancy Gilgoff and he has been teaching worldwide in over 40 countries, since 1979. An accomplished musician, songwriter, film maker and activist, Danny is the first - traveling Ashtanga Yoga Teacher.

Contact: Yogaparadise@yahoo.com / www.dannyparadise.com

David Life and Sharron Gannon- (Jivamukti Yoga) – New York, NY **(9-L)**

Founders of Jivamukti Yoga, Teaching Yoga as a path to enlightenment through compassion toward others.

Contact: www.Jivamuktiyoga.com

David Swenson – (Ashtanga Yoga) - Austin, TX **(9-F, 9-F1, 9-N, 9-O)**

David began practicing yoga in 1969 at the age of 13. His older brother Doug was his first teacher. Then in 1973 David was introduced to Ashtanga yoga when he met David Williams and Nancy Gilgoff in Encinitas, California. Later in 1975 he studied with K. Pattabhi Jois on his first trip to the U.S. and there after on many trips to India.

As one of the few yogis to have learned the original Ashtanga system, in its complete form, author of Ashtanga Yoga the Practice and producer of 8 videos, David has taught this system in 50 countries throughout his 40 years of teaching.

David Swenson is recognized today as one of the world's foremost practitioners and instructors of Ashtanga Yoga. He has traveled to over 50 countries in his 40 years of teaching sharing his knowledge of the system.

Contact: david@ashtanga.net / www.ashtanga.net

Sri Dharma Mittra - (Dharma Yoga) – New York, NY **(9-C)**

Sri Dharma Mittra first encountered yoga as a teenager before meeting his Guru in 1964 and beginning his training in earnest. Sri Dharma founded one of the early independent schools of yoga in New York City in 1975 and has taught hundreds of thousands the world over, in the years since.

Founder of: The system of Dharma Yoga and the (Dharma Yoga New York Center), Worldwide Headquarters. Sri Dharma is the model and creator of the Master Yoga Chart of 908 Postures, the author of *ASANAS: 608 Yoga Poses*, has released two DVD's.

The method of Dharma Yoga has its firm foundation in Yama and Niyama, but gives expression to all eight limbs and nine forms of classical yoga. Sri Dharma continues to disseminate the complete traditional science of yoga through daily classes, workshops and his Life of a Yogi Teacher Trainings, at the Dharma Yoga New York Center and around the world.

Contact: info@dharmayogacenter.com / www.dharmayogacenter.com

---

Jan Thidarat Klinkularb – (Mixed Yoga Styles) – Bangkok, Thailand **(9-Q, 9-W)**

Jan is soft spoken, very kind and has a beautiful Yoga practice. She has practiced and studied yoga with several amazing teachers and has graduated from Doug Swenson's yoga TT program. Now she is practicing and teaching yoga in Bangkok, Thailand.

Contact: ladyjanny@windowslive.com / http://facebook.com/ladyjanny

---

Jonny Kest - (Vinysa Yoga, Yin Yoga and Slowburn) – Detroit, MI **(9-K)**

For over three decades, Jonny Kest has been living the teachings of Ashtanga Vinyasa yoga. His teacher David Williams whom he met at just 12 years old, and his daily Vipassana Meditation practice have been his greatest influences. He believes that the highest form of yoga truly is selfless service. Through continuity, community and compassion Jonny has developed some of the most innovative and evolved Vinyasa Flow practices.

Jonny teaches that *"a posture only becomes a yoga posture when it weakens the tremendous amount of attachment we have in our lives and allows one's own healing power to inspire."*

Contact: WWW.JONNYKEST.COM / DetroitsOriginalVinyasa.com

Joy Kunkanit - (Ricardo and Joy Yoga) – Bangkok Thailand **(9-Z1)**

Joy has studied yoga with Doug Swenson and Larry Shultz and has many years practice in Rocket Yoga and Ashtanga Yoga, Now teaching her own system of Ricardo and Joy Yoga with her husband Ricardo Martin. They are teaching out of Its Yoga in Thailand.

Contact: joykunkanit@gmail.com / www.joyidyoga.com

Kaya McAlister – (Sadhana Yoga Chi & Vinyasa Yoga) Lake Tahoe, CA **(9-E, Pg 215)**

For Kaya, yoga is all about connection and energy. Her yoga practice is about finding a true feeling of unity with the body, mind and soul and with the all-encompassing energy that is Mother Nature. Kaya plans on spending her time traveling the earth, embracing and sharing the benefits of yoga, adventure, and living a healthy life - full of mindfulness and connection.

Contact: kayashannon@yahoo.com, Facebook.com/kayashannonyoga

Yogini Kaliji – (Tri Yoga®) Santa Cruz, CA / International **(9-Z3)**

Yogini Kaliji, the founder of TriYoga, has been guided by *Kriyavati siddhi* to develop this complete method. TriYoga is taught in over 40 countries. Inspired by her love for animals, Kaliji has practiced the vegan lifestyle for 40 years. She is an advocate for the ahimsa trinity of animal rights, human health, and ecology.

Kaliji was conferred the title "Yogini" by H. H. Sri Ganapathy Sachchidananda Swamiji of Mysore, India. In 2006, in recognition of Kaliji's global humanitarian service, Sri Swamiji and Datta Peetham honored her with the Vishwa Bandhu award. Vishnu Bandhu translates as "friend of the universe", a caring relative of humanity. In February 2010 in *Vijaya Karnataka*, Kaliji was called "Great India's Cultural Ambassador." Yogini Kaliji speaks frequently on the ahimsa trinity of animal rights, human health and ecology. Inspired by her love for animals, Kaliji has practiced the vegan plant-based diet for 40 years and has influenced thousands to make healthier food choices.

Contact: www.triyoga.com

Mark Stroud – (World Peace Yoga / Vegan Cooking) – Cincinnati, OH **(9-B, 9-Z7)**

Practicing yoga for over 40 years, Mark is also a Culinary Olympic, award-wining vegan chef, co-founder of World Peace Yoga. He teaches, yoga, cooking classes, philosophy and meditation. Mark was part of the vegan team - at the culinary Olympics in Frankford, Germany, that won a bronze medal.

Contact: yoga@worldpeaceyoga.com / www.worldpeaceyoga.com

Mayra Cadengo – (Sattva Yoga) – Monterrey, Mexico **(9-Z6)**

Founder and Director of **Sattva Yoga®** established in 2002. Mayra teaches many yoga instructors throughout northern Mexico. She started on this path in 1993 and designed the **SMV® Sistema Mandala Vinyasa Yoga.** (Author, Speaker and TV Host) Facilitates yoga and healthy lifestyle in public schools located in deprived areas

Contact: mayracadengo@gmail.com / www.sattvayoga.com.mx

Nancy Gilgoff – (Ashtanga Yoga, Rinzai Zen Meditation) Makawa, Mauai **(9-Z2)**

Nancy began practicing Ashtanga Yoga in 1973 with Sri K. Pattabhi Jois, in Mysore, India. In 1986 she opened The House of Yoga and Zen in Maui, Hawaii where she now teaches daily Ashtanga Yoga classes. She practices (Rinzai Zen Meditation) since 1980 and has studied with Baba Hare Das, along with following the teachings of His Holiness the Dalai Lama. Nancy travels and teaches in the USA, Europe and Asia.

Contact: email address: hyz0@hotmail.com

Paul and Suzie Grilley - (Yin and Anatomy of Yoga) - Los Angeles, CA **(9-X)**

Paul has practiced many styles of yoga since beginning in 1979. His special interest is the integration of ancient energetic theories with modern anatomy and physiology. He Teaches Yin Yoga and Anatomy of Yoga. Paul has published a series of DVD's, including "Anatomy of Yoga" by Paul Grilley. This DVD has given the whole yoga community around the world a fresh new prospective on practicing asana / with many tips on avoiding and over-coming injury.

Paul and his wife Suzie lead regular Yoga classes and seminars for details see the website.

Contact: www.PaulGrilley.com

Ricardo Martin - (Ricardo and Joy Yoga) – Bangkok Thailand **(9-Z1)**
　　　See Joy Kunkanit and Ricardo

Rodney Yee - (Rodney Yee Yoga) – Sag Harbor, NY **(9-P)**

Rodney was a gymnast and a ballet dancer – curiosity lead him to his first yoga class in 1980, which inspired his career and life-long passion as a yoga teacher. The author of 2 books and 30 video titles, Rodney has appeared on Oprah, Good Morning America and a PBS special on yoga. Rodney has been presented regularly in Yoga Journal and in many other popular magazines.

Colleen Saidman - an amazing yoga instructor, yoga celebrity and co-director of Yoga Shanti in Sag Harbor, New York - where she teaches yoga along with her husband Rodney.

Contact: www.yeeyoga.com

Sara B. Turk – (Ashtanga, Sadhana Yoga Chi) – Spring, TX **(Pg 74 / # 5-0, 9-J, 9-Z)**

Sara started vinyasa yoga in the late 1990's, as a complement to her dance training. Since then she has studied meditation, Ashtanga Yoga, Sadhana Yoga Chi and pranayama. In 2010, she opened Cherry Blossom Yoga (Spring TX).   *(Continue Sara Turk on the next page)*

Sara has trained with masterful teachers such as Doug Swenson, Sharath Jois, and Max Strom, who continually inspire her practice and teaching. She shares a successful vegan recipe blog with her sister, the Innocent Primate Vegan Blog, as well as travels teaching workshops and teacher trainings, and assisting Doug Swenson when needed.

Contact: cherryblossom.yoga@gmail.com / www.cherryblossomyoga.com

---

Seane Corn – (Vinyasa Flow Yoga) – Los Angeles, CA   (9-A)

Seane Corn is an internationally celebrated vinyasa flow yoga teacher and thought leader, known for her impassioned activism and unique self-expression, rooted in the themes of self-empowerment, self-actualization and life purpose. Since 2007, through her co-founded organization Off the Mat, Into the World®, Seane and her team have been training leaders in sustainable, authentic activism worldwide, serving underprivileged communities in need.

Contact: www.seanecorn.com

Sharon Gannon and David Life - (Jivamukti Yoga) – New York, NY (9-L)

Founders of Jivamukti Yoga, Teaching Yoga as a path to enlightenment through compassion toward others.

Contact: www.Jivamuktiyoga.com

Shelley Washington – (Ashtanga Yoga – Austin, TX) (9-Z5 / 9-Z8)

Shelley Washington is a legendary figure in the world of Modern Dance. She studied with Twyla Tharp at Wolftrap Academy and American University, prior to being invited to join Twyla Tharp Dance Company in 1975. Previously she danced as a member of the Martha Graham Dance Company. A graduate of Interlochen Arts Academy, Ms. Washington furthered her training at the Juilliard School. In 1977 she performed in the film "Hair" and in 1985 in "singing in the Rain" on Broadway. In 1987 she was honored with a Bessie Award for Outstanding Performance.

In 2000 Shelley initiated her studies of Ashtanga Yoga and dove fully into the practice. She made her first trip to Mysore, India in 2003 and has since made 14 subsequent pilgrimages to Mysore. Shelley received her First Level authorization from K. Pattabhi Jois in 2005 and then received her Second Level authorization from Sharath Rangaswamy in 2010.

Shelley brings a fresh and invigorated energy into the classes she teaches. Her deep compassion, humor, energy, joy and depth of understanding of movement combine to make her a wonderful asset to all of those that have the opportunity to study with her. When not traveling the world Shelley lives in Austin, Texas with her husband David Swenson, their cat, "Yogi" and 15 Koi Fish

Contact: david@ashtanga.net / www.ashtanga.net

Svetlana Panina – (Hatha, Vinyasa Yoga, Yoga Flow) – Moscow, Russia **(9-U, & Cover)**

Svetlana has practiced yoga for more than 10 years, her main focus is in Hatha Yoga and Yoga Flow. In addition to yoga she supports healthy diet and lifestyle. Svetlana's favorite teacher is Doug Swenson and she has assisted Doug for 3 years, with teaching workshops and TT programs in 7 countries. Svetlana teaches yoga classes in Moscow, Russia.

Contact: paninasvetlana79@mail.ru

Tao Porchon-Lynch – (Iyengar based Vinyasa Yoga) - White Plains, NY **(9-T, 9-V)**

Millions across the globe have been inspired by 98-years-young Tao Porchon-Lynch--World War II French Resistance fighter, model, actress, film producer, wine connoisseur, ballroom dancer, and yoga master. Named "Oldest Yoga Teacher" by Guinness World Records in 2012. Starting yoga at age 8, Tao is considered the Grande Dame of Yoga. Her teachers were a Who's Who of the Spiritual World--from the Maharishi to BKS Iyengar and K. Pattabhi Jois. Founder of the Westchester Institute of Yoga in 1982, she has certified over 1,600 teachers.

At the age of 87, Tao became a competitive ballroom dancer and has since won over 700 First Place Awards. She has shared her wisdom at various forums from the Newark Peace Education Summit with his Holiness The 14th Dalai Lama to teaching yoga at the Pentagon and doing a Tedx talk at Columbia University.

Contact: jhpines@optonline.net / www.taoporchonlynch.com

Shri Yogi Hari – (Sampoorna Yoga) – Hollywood, FL **(9-Z4)**

Shri Yogi Hari is a master of Sampoorna Yoga™ (Yoga of Fulness). He is well known and respected around the world as an exeptionally inspiring teacher and Guru. In 1975 he had the blessing of meeting his Gurus, Swami Vishnudevananda and Swami Nadabrahmananda and at that time he retired from the worldly life and spent 7 years in the Sivananda Ashram where he immersed himself fully in yoga sadhana.

Sampoorna Yoga™ is the fruit of Yogi Hari's tireless striving for perfection in his practice and teaching. It is the yoga of fullness that intelligently integrates Hatha, Raja, Karma, Bhakti, Jnana and Nada Yoga. Shri Yogi Hari is the author of 4 books and has recorded over 36 CD's. Regular classes, seminars, sadhana weeks, yoga teacher certification courses and satsangs are given by Shri Yogi Hari at his Ashram in Miramar, Florida.

Contact: www.yogihari.com

PART THREE

Finding Balance

For Health and Happiness

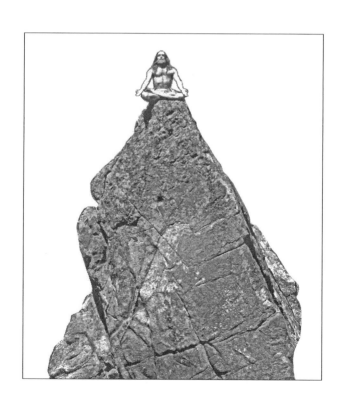

CHAPTER 10

Meditating to Soothe Your Soul

The quiet mind of a yogi

Seeks the answers of the whole universe

The answers of the whole universe ~ Seeks the tranquility of the quiet mind

Meditation is a multi-purpose tool with many wonderful benefits. It releases stress and tension, helps you become more organized, and at the same time assists to create harmony within. The benefits of meditation affect your external life as well. Outwardly you will generate energy with a focused soothing touch, yet remain confident and strong.

You may associate meditation only with monks, nuns, sages, and yoga teachers, but the reality is people of all walks of life are meditating, including the postal worker, secretary and dishwasher, the bank vice president, super model, and of course, yoga students too. Anyone and everyone who wants to improve the quality of his or her mind and life is trying meditation.

In this chapter, I will clearly define meditation and its roots, along with options for various different techniques and some helpful tips- for assisting you with popular aspects of meditation exercises.

Many think of meditation as the absence of thought. However, nothing could be further from the truth. In meditation, you are eliminating the clutter in your head as you discipline your mind, resulting in concentrating your internal power into a very organized and focused resource. Meditation is the means by which you can calm your restless mind until it becomes still, and then focus all your energy and attention on one thought, or area.

Meditation is therefore not the goal, but only a tool that helps you connect to the vital life force. Through meditation you are essentially training your mind to work in harmony with your body, allowing you to reach your full potential.

The Roots of Meditation

Meditation is an ancient art practiced by many cultures and faiths. Many world religions have used meditative techniques, but meditation in itself is not a religious or faith-based activity. Think of it as a mental exercise to help get your mind in shape. What you choose to do with your rejuvenated thoughts are up to you.

For example, Native American shamans, or healers, reached enlightened states through drumming, chanting, dancing, healthy diet and meditation. These activities often led them into a higher level of awareness which lasted for hours or even days. During this enhanced state the shamans were in touch with the vital life force energy, and found a greater connection with the power and softness of nature. They often had visions that inspired them to seek medicinal plants for healing.

Meditation is also a popular technique among Buddhists and is said to have been used by Buddha himself. After Buddha had practiced a restrictive diet, simplicity of lifestyle, and different techniques of yoga for many years, he felt he had looked everywhere for enlightenment to no avail. He realized he had overlooked the inward path, and began to practice meditation. Later, he spent seven days and nights observing his mind while in a constant meditative state. When he emerged from his meditative state he understood the nature of existence, and therefore, was named "the awakened one," or Buddha.

In yoga practice, meditation is one of the eight limbs along the path to enlightenment. Practiced by itself, meditation is called Raja Yoga. In Sanskrit, *raja* means "king," and *yoga* means "union." Raja Yoga therefore translates to the quest to become king of your mind — to focus, tune, relax and control it — while working in unison with your physical body.

The traditional term for meditation is *bhavana*, which translates as "mental and emotional development." Just as you can develop your body through physical exercise, you can develop your mind through mental exercise. Once you have a more focused mental power, you can begin to work on strengthening your emotional development. Experienced yogis and yoginis have more control over their emotions. Showing emotions is not a bad thing, yet there are times when control can produce a positive reaction and become a grand asset to communication.

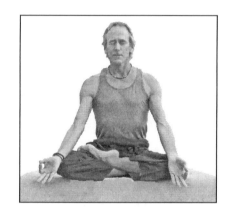

THE FIVE SENSES OF MEDITATION

(Sound, Sight, Touch, Aroma and Taste)
Categories for Meditation

1) SOUND MEDITATION

Repeating a meaningful word or saying: Many people like to meditate using a mantra, which is the repetition of a single word or phrase. Some use the word OM (pronounced *aum*). This word is significant as it symbolizes our connection to the infinite universe. You may want to create a mantra that is meaningful to you. Try something simple, such as "health is wealth," or "kindness speaks through its actions." Some students like to concentrate on ideas they want to manifest in their own personal lives, perhaps something like "strength through softness."

Chanting: Many religions use chanting, or singing as a means of clearing the mind and connect with the power of the universe. If you don't know any traditional chants about gods, saints, or sages, you can make up your own. Try listening to one of the recommendations for chants, you will find listed on the resource page, or pick your own relaxing music which has a similar effect.

You'll know when you've chosen the right music when you hear something that instantly makes you happy. Try meditating on this.

Soothing Music: You may choose to mindfully listen to background music and meditate on the vibration of sound and melody. For newcomers to meditation this is often an easy way to get started, as long as the music does not distract from the meditation.

Sounds of Nature: You may choose to meditate on the many sacred sounds in nature. To mention a few, try focusing on the following: the melody of the wind, or sounds of the distant ocean, the beautiful songs of birds, or the distant echo of thunder. Within nature there are seemingly endless options.

2) SIGHT / VISUAL MEDITATION

Gazing at a photograph, drawing, inspirational image, or nature scene: Gazing at an image is a nice meditation technique. Color, depth of field, and meaning are all important aspects in choosing an image. For example, viewing photographs of nature, or a personally significant work of art can set a tone for successful meditation. If you are lucky enough to be able to meditate outside, you can gaze at a soothing landscape. If you are looking at a picture of a saint, sage, or religious object, you may find that it will help you create a spiritual connection. Whatever you choose, gaze at the image for a few moments, then close your eyes and calmly try to recreate this image in your mind.

Creative Visualization: Many people meditate by visualizing an object that is not actually present. Think of something meaningful to you, and in your mind, place it on a table in a room with nothing else in it. Focus on the color, shape, texture, and smell of the object and allow your other thoughts to float away. Visualization can give your meditation a focal point and help you to calm all the chatter in your mind.

Visualize yourself in nature: One of my favorite techniques is to imagine lying in a beautiful meadow of flowers, on a deserted tropical beach, or perhaps on a mountain top. Imagine you are staring up at white, windswept clouds, and the air is laced with the exotic essence of springtime flowers. In the distance is the soothing sound of a quiet stream.

Experience the moment: If you choose to meditate outdoors, you will experience something wonderful. Whether you are sitting in a beautiful park, resting by a waterfall, or watching a sunset, you are taking time to enjoy the sounds, beauty or silence of nature's soothing touch. Observe all the rich stimuli in your environment and all the sensations in your body; savor the golden moments like a precious love.

3) MEDITATION OF TOUCH

Many people have found the sense of touch to be an excellent focal point for meditation. You may choose from several options using touch as a focal point. Pick a location for your meditation, preferably in a comfortable, clean and relaxing environment. You may practice inside or outside.

3-A) Touching another person, or being touched.
This can be a business massage, touch of friends, or lover.

3-B) Touching non-humans, or objects of nature.
Take your pick from: flowers, tall grass, or rocks by the water, the gentle breeze, sunshine, or sand- you choose.

(Choose your format; and remember if you are outdoors be prepared for changing weather).

Try one of the following techniques:

1. Sit at the base of a large tree on a nice comfortable day, close your eyes and feel the touch of the wind.

2. Walk barefoot in a quiet stream.

3. Touch the silky softness of a flower pedal.

Try one or more of these techniques, with eyes closed or open; and let your mind surrender to the simplicity, gratitude, and very essence of touch.

4) AROMA MEDITATION

As another option, many people have found the sense of smell to be an excellent focal point for meditation, you may choose from several options using aroma as a focal point.

> **A - Aromatic oils for meditation.**
> This is a great way to create the atmosphere for meditation.

> **B - Smelling objects of nature.**
> This is a good excuse to go into nature and create gratitude and awareness of smells.

Essential Oils for Aroma Meditation:

(a) **Frankincense**: promotes deep breathing, allowing for a calmer, deeper meditative state.

(b) **Rose Maroc**: encourages creativity and feelings of love, both for the self and others. This scent also assists in visualization techniques.

(c) **Lavender:** relaxes and balances the mind.

(d) **Rosemary:** promotes mental clarity (and also blends well with Lavender).

(e) **Cedar-wood:** relaxes and calms the mind.

Meditation Environment:

Pick a location for your meditation, preferably in a comfortable, clean, and relaxing environment. You may practice inside or outside.

Meditating with the Outdoors / Try the following techniques:

a) Walk onto a spring meadow and find a nice place to sit. Close your eyes and smell the aroma of flowers.

b) Pick a fresh peach off the tree and smell the rich aroma.

c) Open your window to smell the distant rain or the ocean.

d) Smell the aroma of your favorite food or drink.

e) Try one or more of these techniques, with eyes closed, or open; and allow your mind to surrender with the gratitude, and essence of smell.

5) SENSE OF TASTE MEDITATION

Many people have found the sense of taste to be an excellent focal point for meditation. You may choose from several options using taste as a focal point. Pick a location for your meditation, preferably in a comfortable, clean and relaxing environment. You may choose to practice inside or outside.

a) Savor the flavors in prepared meals and beverages, in fresh fruits and herbs.

b) Try wild berry picking, or harvest other wild foods and savor the very essence of the flavors, as you chew your food well.

c) Enjoy the simplicity of tasting a spice, or one food you enjoy.

d) Taste the essence of a flavorful fruit juice, smoothie, or herbal tea.

Try one or more of these techniques, with eyes closed, or open; and allow your mind to surrender with the gratitude and essence of the flavor.

TWO GUIDED MEDITATION EXERCISES

Below I have listed, two step-by-step guides to get you started on your journey. The first exercise is a basic meditation visualization to help you release stress and tension, and enhance your mental state of mind.

With meditation, the saying, "the journey is everything" fits very appropriately. Along the path of gaining control over your mind, you can strive to practice the following pre-meditations.

A) FIRST MEDITATION TECHNIQUE

(Seated or Laying Down Meditation)

Instructions:

1. **Meditation Posture:** Begin by choosing a comfortable yoga seated posture, such as kneeling pose (Thunderbolt), basic cross legged, Perfect Posture, *Siddahasana*, or half and full lotus *Padamasana*. Refer to Chapter 4 for details on these postures.

2. **On Dwelling:** Try not to dwell on every thought which comes into your mind, instead discard the ones of lesser value.

3. **Redirecting Your Thoughts:** You can take your mind off negative thought, such as hate, worry, fear, and anxiety simply by choosing to think of something more productive.

4. **Embrace Relaxed Yoga Breathing:** Start breathing through your nose as slow and deep as you can; bringing focus to your breath so your mind begins to relax. Make yourself comfortable, think passive thoughts and try to let go of tension in your mind. Completely fill your lungs on inhalations and completely empty your lungs on exhalations. Now incorporate your *ujjayi* controlled sound breathing, gently squeezing the air with your throat muscles, allowing yourself to control the entire duration of the inhalation *and* exhalation.

5. **Progressive Deep Relaxation:** Visualize different areas of your body, starting at your feet and progressing toward your head. Try to suggest relaxation to each specific body area. Try to connect your breathing with your progressive relaxation. As you exhale, isolate each area of your body and visualize it in a relaxed state.

6. **Practice Sense Withdrawal:** Turn your thoughts inward and block out any distractions. This is a major part of the controlled discipline of yoga practice. Try to focus your external thoughts by bringing attention to your posture, breathing, and passive attitude.

7. **Direct your Concentration:** Visualize a flower that appeals to you; explore every aspect of this planet, including its texture, color, fragrance and beauty. Try to recapture this flower in your mind. Its completely normal if the picture fades and other thoughts enter.

8. **Refining your Thoughts:** Simply meditation on the flower. Relax and refine your thoughts to a simple meditation on a flower. Start at the roots of the flowering plant and try to mentally touch the roots in every detail within your mind. Bring your attention up to the stem of the plant, notice the texture. Turn your attention toward the leaves and

notice all the veins running through the leaves. Mentally move to the flower in full bloom, being aware of the beautiful colors, smell its essence and touch the delicate, velvety petals with your mind.

9. **Fading Thoughts:** Allow your thoughts of the flower to fade, and visualize yourself seated in a meadow full of springtime flowers. Listen to your quiet breathing and imagine the softness of the warm evening sun shining gently on your back. Smell the passionate fragrance of springtime flowers riding the soft evening breeze. Bring your thoughts back to the flower and realize that you, the flower, and the whole universe are part of the same energy. Still your mind, quiet your focus and enjoy some moments of peace.

10. **Transcendental Path:** Calmly travel this path as long as you like. When you are finished, relax, clear your mind and sit quietly for another ten, slow deep breaths. When finished lay on your back and relax for few more minutes, then slowly return to your daily activities.

B) <u>SECOND MEDITATION TECHNIQUE</u> - *(Moving Meditation)*

Moving Meditations: A Moving Meditation can be achieved during any movement, such as mindful walking, dancing, surfing, or any other activity, by simply embracing awareness with relaxed mental focus.

> ➤ **B-1: (WALKING MEDITATION)**

To get the most out of this wonderful experience you might first try this walking meditation with a friend for moral support. Find a place to walk and then follow a few simple rules: no talking, and try to embrace action without attachment.

Instructions:

1. **Walking:** Start with yoga breathing- striving to embrace every aspect of your breath.

2. **Adopt the Eyes of a Child:** Be totally aware of every sound, sight, and smell. Pretend you are a small child and have never been out of the house. Experience each moment as if this were your first day on Earth. Find pleasure like never before, from the scent of a flower, be thrilled at the sight of an unusual car, or find detail within unique people.

3. **Reflect and Find Peace:** After 30 – 40 minutes, return home, and sit down trying. Notice if you were aware of your own body and mind, not just outward stimulation. When finished, take some notes and then another day give the Meditation Walk another try. Strive to be aware of every aspect of your own body and mind, yet totally aware of all that is going around you and at the same time be relaxed and at peace.

> ➢ **B-2: (TRISTHANA METHOD) - VINYASA MEDITATION**

A moving meditation can be achieved; by linking yoga asana with a vinyasa, as you embrace total awareness, moving in harmony. This technique will create the ultimate yoga experience, which embraces both the soothing touch of softness and the powerful energy of strength.

Instructions:

As you gain confidence, strength, and greater awareness, you will strive toward having a pure mind-body focus in all aspects of your movements with effortless fluidity and grace. Your practice will float like a cloud, directed by the energy of the wind. At this point you will let your mind flow free, visualizing where you are going with your movements, as your body follows your mind's lead with effortless silence.

Photo Art ~
Doug Swenson &
Kristin Jones

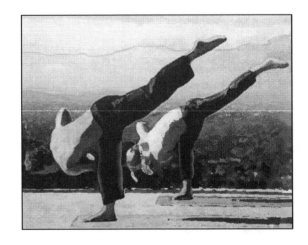

CHAPTER 11

———

Pranayama

The Science, Art and Practice

Energy is life, a sacred design
Like beads of a necklace, prana is sublime

The yoga tradition includes a much focused breathing system that can, in essence, connect your body and mind to the energy of the universe. In fact, yoga gives you all these things and more. Imagine being able to better use your breathing to find greater power, deeper relaxation, enhanced energy, mental clarity, and awareness. This is *pranayama*. In this chapter, you will learn its benefits and philosophy, along with helpful suggestions, precautions and specific techniques.

The word *prana* refers to the vital life force, energy, or power current that runs through all living beings, and the word *yama* means to lengthen. Thus, *pranayama* refers to the electrical current of energy that extends through all of life. The simplest way to think of pranayama is that it is yoga breathing with awareness. When you practice pranayama during yoga, you are striving to be in complete control of the science, art and practice of breathing, and to embrace conscious awareness with every inhalation and exhalation. Prana represents all of the elements of life — earth, air, fire, water, and ether. Yoga practice helps you extract these elements from nature, which replenishes the prana energy in your own body.

The Benefits of Pranayama

In the Hathayoga Pradipika it states, "When prana moves, chitta (mental force) moves. When prana is without movement, chitta is without movement."

In our daily lives, most of us tend to take very shallow breaths. Over time, this incomplete breathing can reduce our overall health and vitality. Yoga breathing is quite different from regular breathing. By consciously making an effort to maintain correct breathing, we are rewarded with more energy, less stress, and better mental focus.

With each breath, you will better oxygenate your blood, muscles, and brain. You will expand your lungs, greatly increasing their capacity and ability to fuel your body. In addition to creating energy, the slow rhythmic, deep breathing in Sadhana Vinyasa Yoga generates a calm, yet focused mind, in both practices, of hard and soft flow, as well as in everyday life.

Studies have indicated that the practice of pranayama helps strengthen the heart, relieve pain, ease cardiovascular and nervous system disorders, and build energy reserves. Through the practice of pranayama techniques, you will release stress, create mental clarity, gain energy and enhance your overall health, plus much more.

THE FIVE PARTS OF PRANAYAMA

Pranayama consists of five parts, each with a different movement, direction and function. The five parts are Prana, Apana, Samana, Vyana, and Udana. According to the teachings of yoga philosophy, all are contained in a sheath called the Pranamaya Kosha, which consists of roughly 364,000 *nadis* (subtle nerve channels) that are connected to other gross and subtle bodies and sheaths.

(1) **Prana:** Literally meaning "air flowing forward," *prana* governs the flow of energy from the head down to the navel, the pranic center of the physical body. It is responsible for all types of inward reception, from inhalation, eating and drinking to the reception of sense perceptions and experiences. Propulsive in nature, it sets and guides things in motion, thereby governing the basic energy that sustains our lives.

(2) Apana: *Apana* means "regressing air" and, like its name suggests, flows downward and outward. It governs the movement of energy from the navel down to the root chakra and is responsible for all forms of systemic discharge, including carbon dioxide in the breath, stools, urine, semen, menstrual fluids, and the fetus. On a deeper level, it forms the foundation of our immune system and governs the expulsion of all negative sensory, mental and emotional experiences.

(3) Samana: Meaning "balanced air," *Samana* flows from the perimeter to the center, in a judicious churning movement. It channelizes the flow of energy from the entire body back to the navel. Primarily it governs the gastrointestinal tract, facilitating the digestion of food and absorption of oxygen in the lungs. Mentally, it serves to digest and assimilate all sensory, mental and emotional inputs.

(4) Vyana: *Vyana* means "air flowing outward." Contrary to *Samana*, *Vyana* governs the conduction of energy from the navel to the rest of the body. Flowing from the center to the periphery, it governs all circulatory functions and assists all other Pranas. It regulates the flow of oxygen, nutrition and water throughout the system, as well as disseminates our thoughts and emotions.

(5) Udana: *Udana*, or "upward moving air," literally moves upwards. It governs energy from the navel to the head. It is responsible for growth, and aids and abets all bodily effort, enthusiasm and will, including the ability to stand and speak. It is the main source of our positive energy in life; *udana* facilitates development of our subtle bodies, as well as evolving consciousness.

Six Cautions for Pranayama Practice

1. In pregnancy, women should not hold their breath or practice rapid, harsh breathing.
2. Children should be at least 5 years old before beginning pranayama practice, and then practice should be moderate.
3. Rapid and vigorous breathing of Kapalbhati **(page 261, # 4),** should be done with caution or avoided if students are post-natal or have the following problems: Abdominal wounds, recent surgical operations, hernia, appendicitis, or a prolapsed rectum or uterus.

4. Students with high blood pressure should get permission from their doctor, yet can generally benefit from light and easy practice.

5. If students have hypertension or asthma, they should not use breath retention.

6. If you feel tired or dizzy, relax into savasana and continue later on or the next day.

The Four Structures of Pranayama:

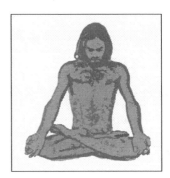

1) - Puraka (controlled inhalation)

2) - Abhyantara Kumbhaka (holding breath in)

3) - Rechaka (controlled exhalation)

4) - Bahya Kumbhaka (holding breath out)

The Two Philosophies: There are two schools of thought, relating to basic techniques of yoga breathing. Both methods are appropriate, as you may find out for yourself in practice.

(1) Three-part diaphragm breathing, or low breathing

Low breathing refers to focusing primarily on the lower part of the chest and lungs. It consists of moving the abdomen in and out with the breath, and changing the position of the diaphragm through these movements. Because of this, it is sometimes called "abdominal breathing." In this type of breathing, you can think of breathing in three parts: expanding the lower abdomen, then expanding the middle of the chest, and then follow with expanding the upper chest.

(2) High breathing, or rib cage breathing

High breathing refers to what takes place primarily in the upper part of the chest and lungs. This technique is often called "collarbone breathing" and involves raising the ribs, collarbone, and shoulders. In this type of breathing, some systems also teach the student to keep their abdominal muscles firm as they expand through the ribs and chest.

SEVEN PRANAYAMA BREATHING EXERCISES

There are many different pranayama exercises described in the Vedas and all will have productive benefits. In this section, I have chosen 7 pranayama exercises which create a nice balance and fit in well with the Pioneering Vinyasa Yoga Program.

1. Basic Yoga Breathing
2. Dirga
3. Anuloma Viloma
4. Kapalabhati

5. Ujjayi
6. Bhramari
7. Simhasana

SEVEN BREATHING EXERCISES / THE INSTRUCTION:

(1) Basic Yoga Breathing

This is a great place to begin exploring pranyama during yoga practice. Basic yoga breathing has three distinct characteristics:

A) - Complete Breathing: For each breath, completely fill your lungs with air on inhalation (*puraka*) and completely empty your lungs on exhalation (*rechaka*).

B) - Slow Breathing: Your breathing is slow, steady, deep, and rhythmic. This controlled breathing enables you to take more oxygen into your lungs, leaving you feeling refreshed and invigorated after practice. It also creates a calm and relaxed mind.

C) - Audible Sound Breathing: The specific technique for basic yoga breathing is called *ujjayi*, which translates as "victorious breath." It involves breathing through the nose with the throat slightly constricted. As you inhale and exhale evenly, the air makes a soft, hissing sound on the back of your throat. This tranquil, meditative sound, in combination with your slow, deep, and calculated breathing pattern contributes to enhancing your energy, calming your body and mind, and enabling you to center your thoughts on your practice.

(2) Dirga (Belley Breathing)

Dirga means "slow, deep long and complete." This technique focuses on breathing into three distinct parts of the body. The first is the belly, on top of or just below the navel. The second is the chest (thorax or rib cage) and the third is the clavicular region or upper chest, near the sternum. As you become familiar with this technique, it is helpful to place your palms on your chest and abdomen to feel the movement of air.

Instructions:

   a) Sit in *sukhasana* or any other comfortable position with back, spine, and neck erect. Alternately you may even lie down on your back. Start by taking slow, long, deep nasal breaths.

   b) As you inhale, let your abdomen fill with air. As you exhale, let your belly deflate like a balloon. Repeat the exercise a few times, keeping your breath smooth and relaxed. Never strain.

   c) Breathe into your belly as in Step 2, but also inflate your thoracic region by letting your rib cage open up. Exhale and repeat the exercise a few times.

   d) Follow steps 2 and 3 and continue inhaling by opening the clavicle region or upper chest. Exhale and repeat the exercise a few times.

   e) Combine all three steps into one continuous or complete flow, quietly feeling the waves of breath move in and out, up and down the body.

Benefits: The practice of *Dirga Pranayama* includes correct diaphragmatic breathing, relaxes the mind and body, optimally oxygenates the blood and cleanses the lungs of residual toxins.

(3) Anuloma Viloma (Alternate Nostril)

Anuloma, means "with the natural order," while *Viloma*, means "going against." In this technique, you inhale through one nostril, retain the breath, and exhale through the other nostril in a ratio of 2:8:4. In yoga philosophy, the left nostril is the path of the nadi called *ida* and the right nostril is the path of the nadi called *pingala*. If you are healthy, you will breathe predominantly through the *ida* nostril for about one hour and fifty minutes, then through the *pingala* nostril for an equal amount of time, alternating back and forth throughout the day. However, in many people, this natural rhythm is disturbed. *Anuloma Viloma* restores, equalizes and balances this natural rhythm and thus the flow of *prana* in the body.

You control the flow of breath with the *Vishnu Mudra*, using your right hand. Tuck your index and middle finger into the middle knuckle of your thumb, keeping your ring and pinky fingers straight. Then, bring your bent knuckles to your nose. Place your thumb by your right nostril and your ring and little fingers by your left, using each to close alternate nostrils as directed.

One round of *Anuloma Viloma* is made up of six steps, as shown below. Start by practicing three rounds and build up slowly to 20 rounds, extending the count within the given ratio.

Instructions:

   a) Inhale through the left nostril, closing the right with the thumb, to the count of four.

   b) It is not necessary to hold the breath, yet if you choose to do so — closing both nostrils, and hold your breath for a comfortable amount of time.

   c) Exhale through right nostril, closing left with ring & little finger.

   d) Inhale through right nostril, keep left nostril closed with the ring and little fingers.

   e) Hold the breath, or choose not to hold the breath.

   f) Exhale through the left nostril, closing right with thumb.

Benefits:

The exercise of the A*nuloma Viloma* maximizes oxygenation of both hemispheres of the brain allowing them to function properly- balancing the left side, which is responsible for logical thinking, and the right side, which is responsible for creative thinking. Yogis consider this to be the best technique to calm the mind and the nervous system.

(4) Kapalabhati (Powerful Exhale)

Kapal — means "skull" and *bhati* means "shinning"; therefore, *Kapalabhati Pranayama* is - sometimes referred to as "Light Skull Breathing" or "Skull Brightener Breath" or "Skull "Breath." This particular technique of pranayama consists of short, powerful exhales and passive inhales. This *pranayama* exercise, has often been used as a traditional internal purification practice, or *kriya*, that tones and cleanses the respiratory system by encouraging the release of toxins and waste matter.

Instructions: (Practice 15 – 20 breaths; 2 rounds)

   a) Rest your hands on your knees, palms facing down.

b) Bring your awareness to your lower belly. To heighten your awareness, you can place your hands, one on top of the other, on your lower belly rather than on your knees.

c) Inhale through both nostrils deeply - Contract your low belly or use your hands to gently press on this area, forcing out the breath in a short burst. As you quickly release the contraction, your inhalation should be automatic and passive, with the focus on exhaling.

d) Begin slowly, aiming for 15 – 25 contractions. Depending on how you feel gradually lengthen and quicken the pace. Always go at your own pace and stop if you feel faint or dizzy.

e) After the exercise, inhale deeply through the nostrils, and then exhale slowly through your mouth. Depending on your experience level, you may repeat the exercise.

f) **Bellows Breathing**: Use same instructions, only now you will inhale and exhale quickly and strongly with equal pressure on the inhalation *and* exhalation.

Benefits:

Kapalabhati is invigorating and warming. It helps to cleanse the lungs, sinuses, and respiratory system, which can help to prevent illness and allergies. Regular practice strengthens the diaphragm and abdominal muscles. This exercise also increases your body's oxygen supply, which stimulates and energizes the brain while preparing it for meditation and work that requires high focus.

(5) *Ujjayi* (Sound Breathing)

Ujjayi, means "victorious breath." In this technique you will learn to control the volume and pace of air, which will control the mind and thoughts as well.

Instructions:
a) Inhale slowly and deeply through both nostrils, slightly constricting your throat muscles, so you hear the air swirling through your throat and control the volume of air passage.

b) Exhale slowly with whispering sound, contract the air passage to control volume of air.

c) The breathing sound is also used as a meditation.

d) Advanced students can retain the breath at the top — for a comfortable and moderate amount of time. This is one single round of ujjayi pranayama.

Benefits:

Strengthens vocal cords, helps activate the thyroid gland, improves blood circulation, and enhances function of the lungs, chest and throat. It also helps one to gain control over the mind.

(6) *Bhramari* - (Humming Breath)

Bhramari, means "bumble bee breath." In this breathing technique you make a meditative sound, which resembles the distant humming sound of bees.

Instruction:

a) Close both your ears with the thumbs of both hands.

b) Close your Eyes with 1st and 2nd fingers.

c) Now slowly inhale deeply through your nose.

d) Retain your breath for a few seconds, and then exhale slowly through your nose, making a humming sound with your throat and buzz like a bee!

Benefits: Calms the body, relieving stress and can make the voice pleasant and melodious, as it strengthens the vocal cords. Also helps to increase concentration.

(7) *Simhasana* (Lions Roar)

Simhasan translates as meaning "lion" and *asana* means "seat," in this exercise you will show your claws and roar like a lion.

Benefits: Releases tension and stress as it expands the lungs - expelling toxins.

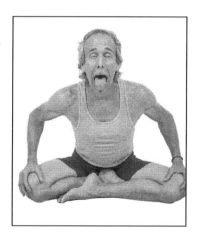

Instructions: (Practice 2 – 3 repetitions, and then relax).

1. Sit on your knees, or cross-legged. Inhale fully, holding your breath for a few seconds, then exhale powerfully, pushing with abdominals and exhale- roaring like a lion.

~ Practicing pranamaya outdoors, in an unpolluted environment. ~
This can be a very inspirational experience.

CHAPTER 12

Discovering Enhanced Diet
For Conscious Yogis

Food of the Gods
Touch the wealth of your soul
Sacred is the mind that can never grow old

You can practice yoga, without any certain diet restrictions, although this concept is very limited in its results and does not represent a holistic approach. In Yoga, and many other philosophies, your body is your temple… to house the sacred spirit and yet many people today, including yogis, treat their bodies like garbage cans. This is true; most people will fill their belly with almost anything as long as it's cheap and tastes good. Unhealthy diets are largely due to lack of education, politics, and a greedy junk food industry. Humans have lost their natural instincts with eating and now rely mostly on cost, advertisement, and peer pressure to make bad choices.

The enhanced nutritional program I teach in this chapter is an education on the highest quality fuel for your body to create abundant energy and mental clarity yet at the same time promotes health and longevity. If that is not enough inspiration, this nutritional program also supports Earth ecology and fuels positive productive thought. All those who adopt this diet program will experience enhanced physical and mental energy, with elevated consciousness and a cool yoga practice too. As an extra added bonus those who embrace these concepts of healthy eating and lifestyle will avoid many negative health issues that plague our modern day society. The foundation to understanding and practicing better nutrition is centered upon first understanding the laws of nature, awareness of food choices and your body's needs.

Laws of Nature and Your Nutrition

I am a firm believer in the philosophy, "health is truly the only real wealth." It does not matter how much money you make, how successful you are, or how famous you become, if you do not have your physical and mental health, the rest holds little or no value.

The importance of proper nutrition is one of the most valuable aspects of this Sadhana Vinyasa Yoga program. Without proper nutrition, you're not going to reach your full potential on any level. Humans are for the most part, in the dark when it comes to nutrition. Throughout time, modern men and women have slowly drifted away from a natural diet and therefore become less healthy, over weight and victims of numerous issues of chronic illness, sickness and disease. Most people today place their trust of healthy diet in the hands of public schools, uninformed doctors and flashy fast food ads with famous athletes. We are further enticed by the marketing pitches, and lured in with tasty and seductive restaurant ads. However, most of these foods are exactly what we don't need to eat. To restore our health and get back on the right path, the solution is simple: Mother Nature knows best.

The good news is that through the Sadhana Vinyasa Yoga nutritional program you can reconnect yourself to the natural flow of energy and the laws of nature, at the same time restoring your vitality and health. This can be done without being totally extreme with: long fasting, shedding your clothes, and living under a rock on a remote mountain, or on a distant planet. You simply have to educate yourself, think sensibly about the food choices you make, and create a plan that puts this valuable aspect of your life into action. Just remember the majority of our society is on the wrong path with nutrition, so you need to adopt will power and a mind of your own.

MOST SICKNESS AND DISEASE / IS DIRECTLY OR INDIRECTLY CAUSED BY:

1. Foods you Eat
2. Liquids you Drink
3. Air you Breathe
4. Thoughts you Choose

Understanding Your Food Choices

All creatures living in the wild, untouched by human civilization, have natural instincts as to what to eat. Each separate species eats the food which is ideal for its own anatomy, health, and well-being. Within each species, the diets of individual animals are almost identical.

Humans, on the other hand, have lost their natural instincts. All of us have basically the same needs for nutrition and yet across the planet we have very diverse eating habits. We'll eat almost anything. The food industry knows if they put something in a colorful box, or serve it in a restaurant with a sprig of parsley, we will eat it, no questions asked! We have completely lost our natural instincts for the ability to make correct food choices. Without this internal guidance system, we can and do choose to eat anything we want, and that freedom can be your friend, or your very worst enemy.

THE GRAVITY OF YOUR FOOD CHOICES

With Six Powerful Reasons for Nutritional Selection

1. Parents and Cultural Heritage

Through destiny, the dice are rolled and you were born into a certain family and culture. Depending on who your parents are and what cultural background they come from will greatly determine the foods we are raised on. As you get older, if you have a mind of your own, this can change. "You are a good Italian boy, eat your pasta!"

2. How Much It Costs

Unfortunately, most of us choose the cheapest food, thinking we are saving money, yet ignoring to add in the eventual extra expense to our health and the environment from eating unhealthy food. "Let's eat at KFC, you get a meal for the whole family — for only $10.99!!!"

3. Easy and Available

Let's face it, most people are lazy by nature, and if food is easy and fast to eat, plus being widely available, then that ranks high with those who only live for today and are not using awareness. "I don't want to drive an extra 5 minutes, just to get healthy food, when I have a cool 7 –11 and Mc Donald's right by my house!!!"

4. Peer Pressure and Fashion

Fashion with; clothes and jewelry, cars and choices of food, all pull heavy gravity in the minds of everyone, because we truly care about the eyes of society and how others see us. Plus, it takes a true individual to ignore the power and influence of your friends, co-workers and mates. "Everyone else in our family eats this way — so what is your problem?" "I worked hard to make your dinner and you are going to get it!!!" "Hey dude, it's not cool to eat kale and apples, we are rock climbers — we live on chicken wings and beer."

5. Enticing Ads on TV, Internet and Print

High tech commercials and ads are designed to captivate your mind and inspire you to buy their products. "Drink at least 3-glasses of milk daily, milk is the foundation of a healthy diet." In time, and with extensive research — many nutritionist and doctors have since proven milk actually causes osteoporosis and a host of many other health issues.

6. Healthy and Nutritional

Sad but true, statistics have proven, most people do not select their food, due to it being healthy. We are in the age of demanding immediate result, and in light of this, very few individuals are looking toward the long term results of diet and lifestyle. This philosophy is also very true in many sports groups, medical drug companies and especially with food providers. Live fast, die young and screw the environment — who cares about the next generation!!!

"You can abbreviate the phrase "Standard American Diet" – **SAD.**

SEEKING YOUR BODY'S ESSENTIAL NEEDS:

First of all, there should be only two classifications of food!

(1) Healthy Natural Foods - (2) Unhealthy Toxic Foods

Unless you are one of the minority, you know: *the health minded person-* you are probably being tempted and greatly influenced to move away from a natural, healthy diet. So in order to enjoy complete health and fill your full potential in all avenues of life, you have to supply your body with certain essential vitamins and minerals that are contained within a variety of unprocessed natural foods.

The Importance of Protein

Protein builds and repairs the body's tissue. Within our body, the basic structure of each cell is comprised of protein. We can get protein from plant or animal sources. Plant sources are preferable for Humans, due to the unusually high fat, cholesterol and bacterial levels in animal products, which have been proven- not be best suited for Humans. Animal sources of protein include meat, dairy, eggs, and fish. Plant sources of dense proteins include nuts, seeds, beans, legumes, grains and spirulina (a fresh water blue green algae and an excellent protein supplement). Other foods containing lower amounts of protein, yet still adding to the daily total are: avocado, cauliflower, collards, garlic, and kale.

FOUR PROFOUND REASONS TO ADOPT A HEALTHY DIET

1. Physical and Mental Health

In today's society we have an epidemic of unhealthy Humans, of which most have slowly drifted away from healthy eating and lifestyle due to lack of education and exploitation of the food industry for profit. This less than healthy society has caused skyrocketing health care expenses, as well as a great loss in one's awareness and mental clarity.

2. Ecology

Eating a poor diet is directly related to pollution of air, water, and land; along with destroying natural resources and wasting of precious water. It might surprise you to know that our fragile environment, in which we all rely on to be healthy and to enjoy life, is very closely associated with the foods which are healthy for us to eat.

3. Animal Cruelty

This means unprovoked killing and needless cruelty of all other living species on this earth. Even if you believe it is your right to torture and abuse all life on this planet, this is definitely not the philosophy of non-violence which is — one of the main foundations of yoga practice. Awareness will teach you that all things are connected with the balance of life and we need every species thriving to insure our own survival. When you destroy and kill nature you are also doing the same to yourself, because you are a part of nature.

4. Logistics of Providing Food

You can feed a vastly greater population on a natural vegetarian, or vegan diet and at the same time exploiting much less of our resources …of water, earth, and air all the while helping to reduce the environmental impact. Fast food, or junk food, might seem like a good idea, because it is cheap, but when you add on the sales tax to your health and the environment, is it then way more expensive.

Traveling the Path to a Healthy Diet:

Nature often gives us warning signals, but we tend to listen to many doctors, who still recommend meat and dairy consumption. Now, members of the National Cancer Institute report that heavy meat eating is related to a high incidence of all types of cancer. In addition, many other experts in the field of nutrition suggest that a diet high in meat and dairy products can actually leach calcium out of the bones leading to osteoporosis. Societies which are mostly vegetarian have a much less chance of getting cancer than meat and dairy consuming societies. Other studies have proven those who base their diet on meat are at higher risk for heart attack, stroke, and artery disease, along with being a host to unhealthy, living practices.

At one time, fish and seafood could have been considered a healthful addition to the diet. However, due to a general lack of respect for nature, many of our ponds, lakes, streams, rivers, and coastal waters are polluted. Therefore, many experts agree it is no longer recommended to eat fish and seafood as a healthy part of good nutrition, unless you are absolutely sure where these foods came from and had them tested for toxins before eating.

The Traditional Yogic Diet
As Listed in Three Food Categories (The Gunas)

Sattvic **Food:** is healthy, wholesome nourishing food. *Sattvic* food supplies your body with all essential ingredients necessary for a healthy active life. These foods would include fresh raw fruits, vegetables, sprouts, nuts, seeds, grains, and sea weed. **(No dairy products – see below)**

Rajasic **Food:** is food that stimulates your body, causing your metabolism and your mind to "run" faster than normal. These foods should not be overused, or they can over-tax your system, which can cause much strain and depletion to both your mental and physical health. This leads to lack of energy, mood swings and over all weakened immune system. A sample of these foods includes coffee, sugar, fructose and herbs such as yohimbi, and ma huang. Through the yogic tradition garlic, onions and spicy foods are placed in this category, only because they tend to unsettle the mind. Garlic, onions and cayenne pepper are very healthy foods though.

Tamasic **Food:** is just plain unhealthy food; eating this kind of food detracts from your health and creates an environment for sickness and disease. These foods include junk food, highly processed food, commercially treated foods, sugar, white flour products, non-organically grown food, fried food, high fat food, meat, dairy products, and eggs.

About Dairy Products and Yoga:
Milk is a part of almost every society, culture and religious background. Even in India's culture as well as its yoga tradition milk has been accepted as a staple. We have all been trained into thinking this is a healthy food. However, humans are still evolving and learning. Also, consider all the recent overwhelming evidence, that proves the inclusion of milk products, after weaning, is counter-productive for a healthy nutritional program and the use of dairy products supports

animal cruelty and abuse. In addition, the use of mass produced dairy products causes' vast ecological devastation. (See "The China Study") For documented for proof!

Think about it, there are no other mammals on this planet that use milk after being weaned from their mother; it is unnatural and totally unnecessary. ***Due to all this evidence you will find I did not list dairy products, under the sattvic food category, of the prescribed yoga diet.***

Choosing Teams and Dancing with the Ego

Regardless of whether you claim the team and badge of being vegan, vegetarian, carnivore, or a junk food junky we should all strive to learn and improve, treating one another with kindness. Look over the priceless evidence in this book and just try a few vegan meals; in the long run you will extend your life and your consciousness, helping to preserve our precious ecological balance of plants and animals. *Awareness and updated education is a priceless gift.* Real Yogi's and yogini's should never close their minds. ☺

Calcium and Protein / Vitamins and Minerals

You will find abundant easily assimilated calcium and protein, vitamins and minerals within; fruits and vegetables, nuts and seeds along with legumes, grains and beans. Experts in the field of nutrition have discovered the diet rich in meat and dairy products actually leaches calcium out of your bones and places you in a much higher risk of cancer, heart and artery disease. (See "Forks over Knives" and the "China Study").

ELEVEN RULES / THE BACKBONE OF A TRUE HEALTHY DIET

To begin your transition, choose one of these rules, and move in that direction. Then try to apply a second, and third. Soon, you will be eating and feeling much better. However, no matter which rule you begin with, try to gradually substitute healthy food and habits with unhealthy food and habits, in addition to cutting back on portions, as overeating is hard on digestion and can be unhealthy for you, even if you are eating healthy natural food.

1) **Base your diet on vegan foods:** then greatly cut back, or eliminate completely all meat and other animal products, including eggs, fish and dairy products too. Eat more fresh raw, steamed, and baked vegetables. Strive for a diet free from all animal products; many experts in the field of nutrition will agree that Humans do not need any animal products to be completely healthy. Use plant proteins; beans, and legumes, with additional protein in nuts, and seeds.

2) **Eat a variety of foods:** and try to avoid eating the same thing every day. A variety of fruits and vegetables, nuts and seeds, beans, grains and legumes — which supply a vast array of healthy vitamins, minerals and essential amino acids.

3) **Eat the rainbow of colors in your foods:** discover that each separate color in foods has a necessary element for holistic health and balanced nutrition.

4) **Reduce the fat:** content in your body, stay away from saturated fats and heated oils. Try to avoid fried foods whenever possible.

5) **Increase the fiber:** in your diet by eating more natural foods, such as; fresh raw fruits and vegetables in addition to whole unrefined grains.

6) **Eat organically grown foods:** Commercially grown food is loaded with chemical pesticides, which are not good for your health or the environment.

7) **Eat more raw plant food in its natural state:** Put more fresh raw foods in your diet. Try to eat whole unprocessed foods. Foods in their whole natural state retain all of the healthy natural fats, carbohydrates, proteins, living enzymes vitamins and minerals as contained in nature.

8) **Avoid over-eating:** especially with rich unhealthy foods and dense proteins - this can cause a strain on the metabolism of your whole body and will greatly shorten your quality of life.

9) **Relax when you eat:** by taking a moment to breathe and appreciate the flavors and colors of our meal.

10) **Add more chlorophyll:** in your diet by eating fresh raw leafy greens, or try green juices and smoothies.

11) **Use a blender and or Juicer daily:** for easy access to nutrients, enhanced health, easy digestion and a natural energy boost.

Chlorophyll / Green Leafy Vegetables and Herbs

The benefits of chlorophyll has been researched and studied for many years in the field of science and nutrition. But what is chlorophyll, what makes it special and what benefits can you get out of it? Listed below, you will be inspired to discover the many wonderful results of using chlorophyll rich foods in your daily diet.

Health Benefits of Chlorophyll

Chlorophyll has been proven to provide many health benefits to those who use it on a regular basis. To begin it has anti-oxidant, anti-inflammatory and wound-healing properties.

1. It has been known to help with the growth and repair of tissues and is very high in calcium.
2. Chlorophyll helps to neutralizing the harmful effects of air pollution, smoking and life in a big city.
3. It efficiently assists to deliver magnesium and helps the blood in carrying the much needed oxygen to all cells and tissues.
4. Chlorophyll is also found to be very useful in assimilating and chelating calcium and other heavy minerals.
5. It has been known to have a great potential in stimulating red blood cells to improve oxygen supply.
6. Along with other vitamins such as A, C and E, chlorophyll has been known to help neutralize free radicals that do damage to healthy cells.
7. Chlorophyll is also an effective way to deodorize and reduce bad breath, urine, fecal waste, and body odor.
8. It may reduce the ability of carcinogens to bind with the DNA in different major organs in the body. Many studies suggest, chlorophyll helps in prevention and overcoming of cancer.
9. Chlorophyll has been used both internally and externally to treat infected wounds.

GETTING STARTED / 3-STEPS FOR SUCCESS

Step One / Planting Positive Thoughts

Choosing to begin a better diet and getting started on a new program of nutrition is the golden first step, for walking the path to a better life. Thoughts are seeds, and if you plant some positive thoughts along the lines of a healthier diet, then these seeds will grow into positive action. Set some time aside, sit down in a quiet place and define your nutritional goals. Do some deep breathing and practice a bit of yoga to enhance your self-confidence. Adopting one new concept is already a major step toward a better life for you and all those you come in to contact with.

Step Two / Building the Foundation

Check the Resource section of this book for suggestions of other books on health and nutrition. Using this information as a guide, make a list of what you need for your new improved diet. Now locate a grocery or health food shop which carries organic natural food. Many supermarkets now have health food sections and a large line of organic products. The cost for natural healthy food may be a bit higher than commercially grown, yet in the long run you will save money on medical expense. Look for healthy alternatives to depleted foods and stock your house with these better foods for your new diet. This will create a positive environment to inspire your succcess.

Step Three / Moving into Action

Put your thoughts and new foods to use by adopting your own level of my healthy diet as suggested in this chapter. Start by substituting one or two healthy meals for your usual meals and remember the best inspiration is to consciously think about what you are eating *before* you eat.

Think about where this food came from, its effects on your body, mind and spirit. Then reflect on our fragile balance of ecology and animal abuse. Try to gradually add more healthy, conscious meals until you have eventually upgraded your whole menu.

"Let your foods be your remedies and your remedies the cure."
— Hippocrates

CHAPTER 13

———

Cleansing with Yoga Kriyas
And Body Detox

Honor thy temple
Cleanse your body and mind
Enticing the spirit divine

Body detoxification is a method to eliminate unwanted toxins and impurities from your anatomy and at the same time greatly enhance the overall condition of body, mind and spirit.

This can be achieved through controlled diet, *Yoga Kriyas,* yoga cleansing techniques, herbs, occasional fasting, and liquid diets consisting of juicing and blending. Body toxins, which accumulate over time through unhealthy diet and pollution, have been proven to be greatly responsible for causing sickness, disease and overall improper functioning of the physical body, which controls our mental functions as well.

The overall focus of this chapter is cleansing the body. For much greater details in an ongoing program to avoid accumulating unnecessary toxins, see Chapter 12 on diet and nutrition.

All of us have accumulated toxins and poisons in our body as a result of the food that we eat, the beverages we drink, the air we breathe and overall exposure to pollution in the environment. Our bodies naturally try to seek out and eliminate unwanted toxins, but our immune systems are outpaced by our unhealthy habits and the massive pollution issues of today. Over time, foreign substances like chemical preservatives, artificial colors, pesticides and heavy metals, along with additional pollutants laced into the air and water, accumulate and slowly weaken our physical and mental body.

There is a natural solution to the complex health problems caused by modern society. The solution is systematic and regular body detoxing, and better food and lifestyle choices. In this chapter you will discover two methods to achieve body detox. The first method uses *Yoga Kriyas,* ancient yogic methods to cleanse the body: and the second uses enhanced diet with an occasional fast from solid food. It is best to incorporate both.

Caution: *Before attempting a body detox it is best to check with a doctor who understands the value of body detoxing, or seek advice from another health care professional. This precaution will help you avoid any unforeseen difficulties.*

A) CLEANSING WITH YOGA KRIYAS

Yoga *Kriyas* are techniques of purification which have been used since ancient times to cleanse the body - not just on the outside, but inside as well.

The word *kriya* by itself means "activity." However, in yoga, *kriya* relates to activity aimed at purifying the mucus membranes of the body. It also includes eye exercises.

Yoga teachers should know that cleaning the outside of the body is just half the job and we should focus on cleansing the filthy insides as well. Most diseases are a result of internal impurities, so to leave this unchecked is a gross failure. Those who practice yoga should be conscious of the fact that to clean just the surface of the body is very much like sweeping dirt under the carpet.

Yoga *Kriya* exercises help to cleanse and detoxify your internal organs, glands, digestive system and skin. Eating healthy food can further assist in cleansing and rebuilding your body and mind form a cellular level, but we live in a polluted environment and even our foods are not as pure as we would like them to be.

The Remedy: Making an effort to do a regular body detox will greatly enhance your body and mind and help prevent sickness and disease.

The Yoga Kriyas are designed to cleanse different areas of the body. Some of these Kriyas are easy to do, and some are better practiced with guidance of a very experienced yoga teacher. In addition, some of the Kriyas are not necessary. In these cases, I have listed a more progressive alternative.

THE SIX MAIN YOGA KRIYAS OR "SHAT KARMA"

1. *Kapalabhati* (Lung Cleanse):

Kapalabhati cleanses the brain and lungs, and can also be used as a specific *pranayama* (breathing exercise). In this technique, you inhale and exhale through the nose, in a short, yet very quick rhythm, for 10 expulsions of air. This fast, rhythmic breathing helps flush toxins from your lungs. When finished, sit calmly for a few slow breaths. (**More details - See Page # 261**)

2. *Trataka* (Eye Cleanse):

This consists of cleansing and strengthening the eyes to improve vision and induce relaxation through eye exercises and washing the eyes. The traditional method of *Trataka* consists of gazing at a candle in a softly lit room, which is cleansing because it allows your eyes to relax and lubricate themselves. To strengthen the eyes you can practice specific eye exercises.

The alternative to candle gazing is to buy an eye wash cup at your local pharmacy and wash your eyes on a regular basis with pure filtered water.

<u>2)-b Eye Exercise:</u> Move your eyes slowly up and down, then close eyes and relax. Now look right to left, then close eyes and relax. Now make circles to the right and then to left, then close eyes and relax. Practice 2 repetitions in each direction, then gently massage eyes and relax.

3. *Nauli* (Stomach Rolling):

This action and control of the abdominal muscles creates an internal massage, cleansing and toning the abdominal organs and intestinal tract and enhancing digestion. In this technique, you roll your stomach like a wave, from right to left. This Kriya is also great for toning the abdomen, and benefits the functions of the liver and kidneys, which are responsible for the elimination of impurities from your body. *Nauli* is achieved by: a) Exhale your air and then lift your stomach in and up, b) Then drop the rectus abdominals (Middle ridge of stomach muscles), and c) Roll your stomach muscles from right to left and then left to right.

4. *Neti* (Nasal Wash):

Neti is a washing of the nasal passages using a warm saline water solution. This *kriya* sounds rather dramatic, but it's really a simple practice. You fill a small pot (known as a neti pot, available in natural food stores and some pharmacies) with warm salt water, then place the pot's spout in your nostril and tip it back so the warm water flushes through your sinus cavity. This *kriya* helps cleanse the sinuses of excess mucus and bacteria.

5. *Dhauti* (Stomach Wash):

*** I do not recommend this Kriya – see alternative method below
Dhuati refers to the technique of washing the esophagus and stomach with water, then inducing vomiting. Ancient yogis devised this Kriya as a means of cleansing the digestive system. **I list it here for your education, but I definitely don't recommend it**, as there are other ways to wash the stomach.

*** A better method is to simply mix the juice of half a lemon and a dash of cayenne pepper in a large glass of warm filtered water, and drink it first thing in the morning before eating solid food. This will cleanse your stomach, kidneys and small intestines and also inspire a bowl movement.

6. *Basti* or *Vasti* (Colon Wash):

This original technique of cleansing the rectum and colon with water is equivalent to the modern day enema or colonic. I strongly recommend that you go to a qualified professional for a colonic, or you can do an enema in the privacy of your own home. Many people find this *kriya* helpful three to four times a year, as a clean colon inspires health and mental clarity and has been proven by authorities in the field of health and nutrition to greatly assist in the prevention and overcoming of some chronic sicknesses and diseases.

B) CLEANSING WITH / RESTRICTED DIET AND FASTING

Authorities in the field of health and nutrition have proven that a low calorie, high nutritional diet coupled with occasional fasting is one of the best ways to help eliminate toxins and restore vibrant health. Juice fasting, blended nutritional smoothies and an exclusive raw food diet, also cleanses the body of excess mucus, stored chemicals, and drugs that will distract from your health, vitality and longevity. Many people try a restricted diet, or fast, for the sole purpose of losing weight, however this is not a recommended solution - as most people find they quickly gain the weight back as they return to poor eating habits.

What Happens to Your Body During a Detox or Fast?

During a conscious body detox or fast, your metabolism has a built-in response to begin searching every part of your anatomy for unwanted toxins and weakened or diseased cells, and to remove them from your blood stream. There are five avenues for elimination: the lungs, kidneys, bowels, mouth, nose and skin. In a healthy body all these avenues of elimination are allowed to operate freely. If any one of these avenues is blocked, your health will be compromised. It is not healthy, natural, or advantageous to keep unwanted toxins from being eliminated from your body. During a fast, or restricted cleansing diet, all these avenues of elimination are greatly enhanced and will help create an easy elimination of toxins from your body.

To Review / Five Avenues to Eliminate Body Toxins

1. Lungs (through exhalation)
2. Kidneys (through urination)
3. Bowels (through stool)
4. Skin (through sweating)
5. Nose and mouth (through mucus discharge)

Caution: *Before attempting a body detox or fast it is best to check with your doctor, or a health professional who works with the laws of nature to insure your health and wellness.*

Levels of Detoxifying Fasts and Diets:

Here, I will share three levels of body detoxes or fasts to embrace a wide range of individuals. Choose one of the following methods that best suits to your own needs, or just eat a strict raw-food diet without any animal products. It is advisable to start your cleansing by washing the impurities out of your colon through the use of an enema or colonic. You can do an enema in the privacy of your own home with a half-gallon of warm water, or look up a colon therapist in your area to book an appointment for a colonic. Either one or both methods will greatly assist in the cleansing process.

Caution: *If you have a blood sugar problem, dilute your fruit juices 50 percent or more with pure water, or substitute with fresh squeezed, green vegetable juice such as celery, cucumber, lettuce and kale. You will also benefit from supplementing your body cleansing with blue-green algae (cyanobacteria) or spirulina.*

ORGANIC VERSES NON-ORGANIC

We should classify fresh produce into the following two categories:

1. Natural Food (Organically Grown)

This is whole unprocessed natural foods, as found in nature – without harmful chemical sprays and toxic fertilizers.

2. Chemically Poisoned Food (Commercially Grown)

It goes without saying we should always try to choose organically grown products, especially when doing a body detox. If you do not choose the organically grown option, you are just putting more toxins into your body and supporting widespread pollution of the environment.

The FDA sets standards for safe levels of toxins in your foods, which allows for certain doses, of toxic chemicals to be allowed in your foods. When you eat non-organic foods you are taking much higher doses of unhealthy chemicals into your body, and supporting the fact that they end up in the soil and waterways of our fragile earth ecology.

A) Start Light Cleansing - (Complete Guide)

This cleansing is ideal for those who have a poor diet and little or no experience with body detoxification. This cleansing restricts your diet to strictly: fresh, raw, uncooked fruits and vegetables with an ample amount of dark leafy greens.

A) <u>Sample Light Cleansing:</u>

If you have blood sugar problems, skip sweet fruit, instead choosing low glycemic fruits like grapefruit or lemon, or substitute by using cucumbers and celery.

<u>For Breakfast</u> -

To Drink:

One tall glass of pure water with juice of ½ lemon; or warm, non-caffeinated herbal tea (try to avoid using sweeteners). Drink liquids 15 minutes before eating, or make a smoothie instead of eating.

To Eat / Blended or Whole:

1 or 2 seeded - fresh, raw and unprocessed fruits.
Seeded fruit is higher in nutrition and lower in sugar than seedless fruit.

Remember: If you have blood sugar problems, skip sweet fruit, instead choosing low glycemic fruits like grapefruit or lemon, or substitute by eating cucumbers.

Do not eat:

Dried fruit, nuts, seeds, grains, animal products, or processed food. These will stop the cleansing process.

<u>For Lunch</u>

To Drink:

One tall glass of pure water with juice of ½ lemon; warm, non-caffeinated herbal tea; or fresh juice diluted with water (try to avoid using sweeteners). Drink liquids 15 minutes before eating or make a smoothie instead of eating.

To Eat / Blended or Whole:

Eat a fresh, raw salad with a variety of vegetables using lemon and ½ avocado for dressing.

Do not eat:

Remember not to eat Dried fruit, nuts, seeds, grains, animal products, or processed food. These will stop the cleansing process.

Dinner

To Drink:

One tall glass of pure water with juice of ½ lemon; or warm, non-caffeinated herbal tea (try to avoid using sweeteners). Drink liquids 15 minutes, before eating, or make a smoothie instead of eating. *(For a deeper cleanse, choose only a liquid meal.)*

To Eat / Blended or Whole:

A small, fresh, raw salad with a variety of vegetables and fruits using lemon juice for dressing or just enjoy without dressing.

Do not eat concentrated foods:

As with lunch avoid dried fruit, nuts, seeds, grains, animal products, or processed food. These will stop the cleansing process.

This light cleansing has no restrictions between meals on pure water, herbal tea, fresh green juices, or snacking on low glycemic fruits, celery sticks and dark leafy greens. Continue this program for 1 to 4 days.

Breaking your Light Cleansing:

Choose your first meals wisely. Eat some lightly steamed vegetables for a few meals, then gradually include nuts, seeds, beans and whole grains. Take steps to adopt a healthy diet. **Do not break your fast with unhealthy foods or drinks. No animal or dairy products, no processed carbohydrates, and no heavy proteins. Avoid overeating. This can greatly undo all the benefits and in some cases be quite dangerous.** It is important that your first few meals after a body detox are very healthy, light and cleansing in nature. For more details, see: "Breaking your Fast." **(Details for breaking the fast - See Pg # 282 and 287)**

B) Start Moderate Cleansing - (Complete Guide)

This is best suited for those who are predominately vegetarian and have tried body detoxification in the past. A moderate cleansing removes almost all solid food from the diet, so that you are blending or juicing only raw, uncooked seeded fruits and fresh raw vegetables (making healthy smoothies, or juices). It is advisable to add lots of green leafy vegetables to your juice or smoothie. Dark greens greatly assist in the removal of toxins, enhance energy, and protect your body from environmental pollution.

Sample Moderate Cleansing:

If you have blood sugar problems, skip sweet fruit, instead choosing low glycemic fruits like grapefruit or lemon, or substitute by using cucumbers and celery.

For Breakfast

To Drink:
Choose one of the following three options.

1) One tall glass of pure water with juice of ½ lemon and a dash of cayenne pepper. This may be warm or cool.

2) Non-caffeinated herbal tea. Try to avoid using sweeteners.

3) A fresh-squeezed fruit and vegetable juice combo, diluted with water.

To Eat / Blended or Whole:
One or two: seeded fresh, raw and unprocessed fruits.

Seeded fruit is higher in nutrition and lower in sugar than seedless fruit.

For Lunch

To Drink:

Drink one tall glass of pure water with juice of ½ lemon; non-caffeinated herbal tea; or fresh mixed fruit and vegetable juice, diluted with water. Do not use sweeteners.

To Eat:

1 or 2 leaves of kale, raw and whole, not chopped.

For Dinner

To Drink: (To Eat / No solid foods / Only Liquids)

Drink one tall glass of pure water with juice of ½ lemon; or non-caffeinated herbal tea. Do not use sweeteners).

This moderate cleansing has no restrictions on liquids between meals, so you can have unlimited pure water, herbal tea, and fresh green juices. **Continue this program for 1 to 4 days**.

Breaking Your Moderate Cleansing

Choose your first few meals wisely. Eat a raw salad and or fresh fruit for your first meal. For your next meal, three hours later, add a raw, or cooked vegetable. Add blended nuts or raw nut butters to your salad and fruit.

Then, gradually adopt a healthy regular eating program. Use lightly steamed vegetables for a few meals, then gradually include nuts and seeds, legumes, beans and whole grains. Take steps to adopt a healthy diet.

Do not break your fast with unhealthy foods or drinks. No animal or dairy products, no processed carbohydrates, and no heavy proteins. Avoid overeating. This can greatly undo all the benefits and in some cases be quite dangerous. It is important that your first few meals after a body detox are very healthy, light and cleansing in nature. For more details, see "Breaking your Fast." **(Details for breaking the fast - See Pg # 282 and 287)**

C) START DEEP CLEANSING - (COMPLETE GUIDE) ON NEXT PAGE

This cleansing is best suited for those who are already vegetarians and striving to become vegans, with at least 70 percent of their diet being raw food. A deep cleansing is considered to be a true fast. It restricts the intake of all solid food, and includes drinking only fresh squeezed diluted fruit juices, diluted vegetable juices and diluted leafy green juices, supplemented with filtered water and herb teas. Green drinks are made of the juice extracted from fresh, raw, chlorophyll-rich vegetables such as celery, cucumber, spinach, lettuce, kale, parsley, and collard greens.

Sample Deep Cleansing

If you have blood sugar problems, skip sweet fruit, instead choosing low glycemic fruits like grapefruit or lemon, or substitute by using cucumbers and celery.

For Breakfast

To Drink: (No Solid Food)

Pure filtered water with juice of ½ lemon and a dash of cayenne pepper. This may be warm, or cool.

For Lunch

To Drink: (No Solid Food)

A freshly squeezed juice of leafy green vegetables and celery with a small amount of apple and ½ lemon.

Dinner

To Drink: (No Solid Food)

Warm, or cool herbal tea for dinner.

This deep cleansing has no restrictions on liquids between meals so you can have unlimited pure water, herbal tea, or fresh green juices. **Continue this program for 2 to 5 days.**

Breaking your Deep Cleansing

Choose your first meal wisely. Eat 1 or 2 pieces of fresh raw seeded fruit and then a raw salad, using lemon for dressing. On the second day you can add avocado and a few nuts. The third day, add lightly steamed vegetables and gradually return to a healthy eating program.

Remember the addition of cooked foods, protein or starch, will partially or fully stop the elimination of toxins and you will no longer be in a cleansing, body detoxification mode. During fasting, your body will rest, cleanse, rejuvenate, and try to heal your whole system naturally. For best results, it is most appropriate to pick a time when you can rest, or at least cut your work and stress load down greatly. Practice light yoga and take easy walks. At night, relax in a warm Epsom salt bath.

Almost anyone can safely fast or maintain a restricted diet for 1 to 3 days. If you are very healthy you can fast up to 5 or 6 days. A fast longer than **3-days is not advisable** without the supervision of a doctor or licensed professional. Again, if you have blood sugar problems, stay away from sweet fruits and vegetables, and dilute your juices.

Preparing for Liquid Diet

It is best to first change your diet before you begin a fast so your body doesn't go into shock. Slowly move away from processed food, junk food, and meat and animal products. Introduce more raw and cooked fruits and vegetables, nuts, seeds, grains, and fresh fruit and vegetable juices. After a few weeks of an improved diet, you can try to fast anywhere from two to four days.

It is advisable to start and finish your fast with an enema or colonic. During your fast, your intestines will become loaded with poisons from the body as your system tries to eliminate these toxins. An enema or colonic will greatly assist in removing this waste from your colon much quicker than your normal metabolic function can and therefore leave you feeling very refreshed.

The Emotional Response to Fasting

The second limb of the eight limbed yogic path to enlightenment pertains to ethics and morals. In particular, only hard work and effort builds paradise. You cannot achieve health by having it handed to you. The Sanskrit word *tapas* translates as meaning "effort or burning," which involves self-discipline, purification and austerity. The word, "austerity", in this context means to work at something whereby there is an exchange between discomfort and attaining a positive goal. *Tapas,* broadly means that you need to undergo some physical and mental discomfort in order to achieve enhanced physical and mental health. While many of us want an instant cure, it is not possible and it does take energy and changing bad habits with conscious good habits to succeed.

Fasting can be very hard work, depending on the level of toxins in your body. While your body is eliminating toxins, you will experience days when you feel dizzy and weak. Other days you will feel on top of the world. It is best to avoid extensive physical and mental stress during your fast. Some people have more energy during a fast, while others will feel weak, drained and emotionally fragile. The slight discomfort is a small price to pay for a clean bill of health.

Extra Notes on Breaking the Fast Early

If you begin your fast and feel like you cannot or do not want to go the distance, simply break your fast by eating sensibly. Your first meal should be a leafy green salad without dressing, or fresh juicy seeded fruits.

The first few days following a successful fast should consist of meals that have a laxative or cleansing effect. The reason for this is that it is very important to quickly eliminate the toxins that have been stored up throughout the body as a result of the fasting or cleansing.

Important note:
When you break your fast, or restricted diet - steer clear of all less healthy food and drinks, avoid over eating, eat slowly and enjoy the simplicity and flavors of your foods.

Yoga Is

an empty cup... just waiting
to taste the richness
of your soul.

Patience, is times wife
so longing to find...
lost thoughts in timid minds,

as another vinyasa wants to Fly.

----Doug Swenson

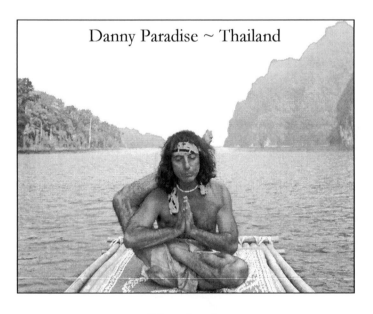

Danny Paradise ~ Thailand

Live simply
So that others may simply live
------ Mahatma Gandhi

PART FOUR

Living the Path
And Evolution of Yoga

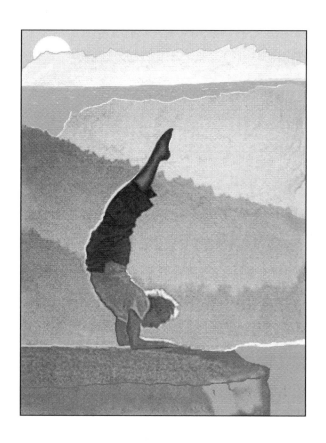

CHAPTER 14

Four Stories
Of the Peaceful Warrior

Our life is often like a movie, as we can look at one frame, or moment, and then find a whole episode waiting to be rediscovered. Some moments from the past may be very heartbreaking or tragic. On the other hand, we recall incidents that reflect happy times with friends, family, or lovers. We remember amazing adventures, or times we found a deep sense of contentment and inner peace.

Sometimes looking back, we embrace rich instances of simplicity to savor as sweet nectar in time. Then we relive experiences where we were being creative and expressing ourselves, which are priceless gifts as we learn the freedom of our true nature. If we reflect on the whole picture attached to every moment, painful or sweet, each is a learning experience as we play our role in the movie of life.

In this chapter, I have chosen four specific episodes along my path to share with you. Each is both personal, as well as a reflection of the evolution of yoga practice in the U.S., and a colorful illustration of how problems are often gifts in disguise.

In hindsight, we see many times when we were trying to move forward but gravity was pulling us back, knowing now those encounters actually served to make us stronger and inspired true wisdom. We all have goals and dreams, yet often we have to overcome challenges to achieve them. With the benefit of time, we realize many of our obstacles did not arise from the others we blame, yet from our own self-ego, which blocked progress.

Here, my four stories await you patiently as the adventure begins.

One Drop of Water
In the Ocean of Opposition

We are all born into this life in different places and specific moments in time.

IT has been said by many philosophers that problems are gifts in disguise, and with this in mind, each challenge becomes a learning experience — that is, for those who have the insight to see the true lesson. As for the others, who are going through life blindly as if they are driving without their headlights on, they will have to wait until they are illuminated enough to realize when another gift appears.

Each circumstance, regardless of its nature — whether it is truly pleasant, or downright difficult — always has a hidden lesson attached, a message for your inner self or those around you.

Our brains are much like computers, as we are programmed to respond to the information we gather and store. We are greatly influenced by our surroundings — relatives, teachers, culture and human society as a whole. Ideally, this programming is given to us as helpful guidelines to teach us right from wrong, and to further develop our mental perception and expand our knowledge.

But this process often gets derailed, because the bulk of society is nervous and frightened when confronted with change, or when experiencing a new and seemingly strange approach to a more progressive life. As humans, a truly priceless gift is the ability to see ourselves and the delicate balance between being programmed like a computer to respond as authorized, or in taking a good look as an individual, to process knowledge into something more progressive or new, thus coming to our own conclusions. Discerning the difference is the foundation to intelligence and awareness. As action creates reaction, karma is born. In the Hindu philosophy, this becomes our resume for future employment on earth.

We should learn to listen to our thoughts, as clouds should listen to the wind — where destiny awaits.

For me, childhood was a total adventure, laced with choices, opinions and unpredictable consequences. But beginning in my pre-teen years, whenever I was presented with a new concept to live by, I began to filter out correct, essential and progressive information from less productive and incorrect information, digesting what I could and passing off the rest.

It was in this way I began to break free of the bonds and cultural heritage of my conservative hometown of Houston, Texas and forge my own path.

But let me start at the beginning.

I was born March 3, 1951 in Houston, Texas. My childhood was really wonderful, especially since my parents Stanley and Violet Swenson were kind, loving and open-minded. Ever since I can remember, I was drawn to past times and hobbies of nature related origins: like building tree houses, riding my bike and playing in the mud. Once my brother David was born, I was totally excited to have a little brother to share my vast knowledge from my five years of experience. Very shortly after David could walk, we started experimenting with skate boarding, building better tree houses and playing in the woods all day long. My big sister Diana was more refined and cultured with interest in dance, fashion and the latest cool, rock bands. On occasion, Diana would help with suggestions to keep David and I from getting in trouble with the parents.

I didn't think much of the wider world until age 13, when I began to question the validity of the lessons I was being taught in school, by my family, and from human society as a whole. I was just not quite sure these lessons were all one hundred percent correct, and, most of all, I was positive there was something missing. I felt there was definitely more valuable information to learn, if I could only find it.

As I woke up to my way of free thinking, my questions, thoughts and fresh new ideas were not always appreciated at that place and time, in the conservative environment that surrounded me. It seemed there were no like-minded souls to be found, and I received constant verbal warnings and cautions for entertaining my foolish insights. After all, what could I possibly know? I was just a kid!

I was very lucky to have a mother and father who were kind, caring and quite open-minded as compared to many of those around us. My parents belonged to "The Unitarian Fellowship," a church group whose members were encouraged to think both inside and outside the boxed and packaged presentation of society.

One Sunday, my parents wanted me to meet an older man who was supposed to be quite interesting. His name was Ernest Wood. This was not the first time I had been introduced to a member of the church group, or to friends of my parents, but it was definitely the most memorable. As I shook his hand, I was immediately drawn to his eyes, the tone of his voice and the energy that embraced his presence. During those few moments I saw something, and it was beyond words to describe, yet my brain became relaxed and my thoughts at peace. Little did I know this man would eventually greatly influence my life in many ways.

The following week, Ernest Wood was asked to teach a class to some of the Sunday school kids. I was one of the lucky ones and curious as to exactly what it was Mr. Wood would teach us. As it turns out Ernest Wood was a published author, yoga master, Sanskrit scholar and philosopher, and he was teaching yoga to us on this day, although I didn't necessarily realize it at the time. The philosophy and metaphors Ernest Wood taught in class were sometimes a bit over my head, but I never forgot the Yoga postures, breathing and deep relaxation along with subtle words of wisdom and the amazing feeling that remained with me after class, which was far beyond any experience I had ever encountered.

I was about to turn 14 and, like most young teenagers; I had many ideas going on at the same time. One of my interests, which ranked at the top of my list, was surfing; being on the ocean, at peace with the world and riding a wave. For me surfing was a truly sacred and spiritual experience! We lived a two-hour drive from the nearest ocean, the Gulf of Mexico, which was definitely not famous for world class waves. I listened to songs about surfing, and saw photographs of distant lands with way cool swells. I knew I would have to convince my parents to give me a ride to the beach now and then, but I was already a good skateboarder and after all, in my way of thinking, water was softer than concrete. My dream became reality when my parents agreed to assist me with the purchase of a surfboard, provided I did well in school, could complete my chores around the house and would work a part-time job to pay my share of the expense.

The thought of having my very own surfboard and learning to surf was worth any effort and energy I had to endure to get there. Six months later, I had reached my savings goal of $55 and upheld my other obligations, so my parents and I went to the local surf shop and purchased my surfboard. The very next weekend I bummed a ride to the beach with my older sister's friends, who were also learning to surf. In the months to come, I found complete bliss in the energy of the ocean, as well as in some of the concepts of breathing, stretching and relaxation that Ernest Wood had taught me. When I turned 15 and started my freshman year in high school, I realized my hobbies of surfing and "Yoga stretching" made me different from the other kids in high school.

One day I was looking at a surfing magazine with beautiful photos of waves in Southern California and I immediately started to spend long hours thinking about how I might convince my parents to allow me to see this surfing paradise. I got my chance when my sister's older boyfriend Gary bought a car. He was also a surfer, as well as a smooth talker, and after several attempts Gary convinced my parents to allow me to travel with him to California for three weeks that summer. All went well and I found myself surfing a wonderful and really magical spot rightfully named Swami's. At the time I did not connect the dots, but the next day when I came in from the ocean I noticed a beautiful building perched on the cliff above Swami's surfing beach. Curious, I walked by the grounds and noticed some people doing a few of the movements Mr. Wood had shared. I quickly ran over and ask just what this interesting technique was called?

"We practice yoga, this is an ancient and sacred mind-body philosophy," they replied.

A light turned on in my brain as I realized what Ernest Wood had taught me, those years before, was yoga practice and philosophy. Being young at the time I did not understand the full impact of what he was teaching me until that very moment, standing on the grounds of what I was then told was the "Self Realization Fellowship" founded by Paramahansa Yogananda. I went inside the temple and had a wonderful vegetarian lunch.

After another five days of surfing it was time to return home to Houston. As soon as I walked in the door I told my father I wanted to do more yoga with Mr. Wood. My father gently told me Mr. Wood had recently passed away, but that he had three of his yoga books, which he proceeded to share with me. In the year 1965 in Texas there were no yoga studios and I did not know of one other person practicing yoga. So, Ernest Woods's books became part of my regular studies, along with my school textbooks, and of course, surfing magazines.

In time, I began to learn about the benefits of a healthy diet, and as I continued to adhere to regular yoga practice my surfing excelled beyond all of my wildest dreams. Yet all was not well. In school I was constantly bullied for being a "surfer, yoga dude and vegetarian weirdo." As I was heckled, I escaped with thoughts about surfing and dreams of moving to California, where people with my beliefs and passions were commonplace. In the meantime, my parents were encouraging me to work a good job in Houston and to cut my hair in order to look presentable and more appropriate.

As the pressure to conform built up and became unbearable, at the age of 17, I decided to leave home and move to California against my parents' wishes. Due to my parents' concern, they sent me to three psychiatrists, who only served to unintentionally confirm my reasons for leaving. I had friends in Encinitas who agreed to rent me a room. I arrived in 1968 and enrolled in the local high school, telling them I had moved there with my parents. For money, I worked after school at Ocean Pacific Surf Shop where I made surfboard wax and did some janitorial duties.

In a very short time, my surfing and yoga excelled to a level which was off the charts. OP sponsored me as a professional surfer, and I did so well I went on to compete throughout the U.S. and around the world, including the 1972 world surfing championship in Oceanside, CA. My yoga gave my surfing a turbo boost and a peaceful and relaxed relationship with the ocean, while the waves enhanced my yoga by teaching me about the movement of energy and the value of cross-training, both physically and mentally.

I never really thought about teaching yoga until my fellow surfers started asking if I might share this magic and priceless gift. I agreed, and held my first 'class' in 1969. I had progressed from being bullied in school to being a rock star surfer and a highly respected yoga teacher. The not-so-easy days of being raised in Texas had ironically taught me to be strong, to have faith in my dreams and to stand my ground even when faced with endless opposition in all directions. Now I was living in California with like-minded souls, surfing, practicing yoga and eating an enhanced vegetarian diet with endless energy and mental clarity.

The strongest Human is the one
With the greatest strength of progressive thought
In the midst of vast opposition

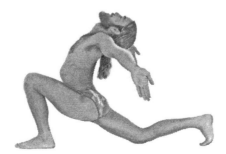

Being Prana
The Essence of all Life

At age 23, after I had been practicing yoga for 10 years, this mystical practice was finally being acknowledged in many parts of the U.S. and around the world as a powerful tool to enhance physical and mental well-being, as well as cultivate inner peace.

Society was slowly becoming more familiar with the amazing benefits of the sacred science and art of yoga. I decided to take a month or so, to do some informal experiments with practicing yoga in various environments, both indoors and outside with nature. The results were quite amazing. When I practiced outdoors, the benefits were greatly multiplied and I discovered amazing rewards I never before experienced.

In my first experiments, I picked a nice, quiet park with lots of green grass and shady trees, and not too many bugs. This was an easy introduction to outdoor practice. The most important thing was being surrounded by the living energy of plants, which were oxygenating the air. After every outdoor practice my eyes were clear, my mind embraced a much deeper sense of inner peace, and I had a glow to my presence. These results were at a level I had never before noticed with indoor yoga practice, and I was inspired to try more outdoor sessions.

As I gained more comfort with further practice in nature, my mental states began to travel farther beyond the norm, and I found myself becoming much more intuitive, with a greater sense of awareness, compassion and mental focus. These results were not just confined to the time and particular location where I practiced on any given day, but stayed with me at work and home, sometimes lasting six hours or more. On many occasions after I had an amazing outdoor practice, people I came in contact with throughout the day commented that they felt at peace just being in my presence.

Imagine walking into a room full of negative, unproductive, low-energy people — the type who see the cup half empty and look for reasons to complain, dragging everyone else into their dark space like the black hole of a fallen star that sucks everything into its void.

Well, after a great outdoor yoga practice, I was glowing with the opposite effects, and as I absorbed the power and softness of the whole universe I found I could lift people out of black holes, depression and dark thoughts, all without saying one word. The credit was not mine to own. It was not magic, nor did I have secret powers. Yet I found a way to channel the incredible presence of nature through outdoor yoga. With immense prana as my companion, good things began to happen.

In the next month or so, I began to notice nature at a much deeper level, such as the way the wind blew through the trees, the power and softness of the river, the strength of the mountain and tranquility of the sunset or sunrise. I observed, more intimately, the way oceans changed into clouds, then became rain or snow and finally returned to the sea. I realized yoga was teaching me lessons on how to have faith in invisible energy, how to float like the wind. It was teaching me to embody the fluidity of a river and the power of a mountain, and to be inspired by the way the ocean changes and creates life. Yoga allowed me to be the light and tranquility of the sunrise and sunset.

I learned priceless information and much more which cannot be easily explained in words.

Practicing outdoors at sunset also led me to my first discovery of *vinyasa*, defined as the connecting link between yoga postures. In order to get a visual of what I was doing, I watched my shadow as it moved over the ground. When the shadow drew smooth, flowing energy lines, I noticed my practice felt better, and this translated into more fluid and productive actions throughout my daily life.

In addition to instilling increased mental clarity, peace, compassion, strength and spirituality, there is one more quite interesting aspect of outdoor yoga practice: The Law of Attraction.

I discovered I would often attract animals, birds and reptiles which seemed to feel at peace in my presence. They watched me and communicated without words. When I was deep into my asana practice, these creatures accepted me. It was as if they praised me for not being noisy, violent, or afraid and for blessing their space with kindness and love. They respected me as I learned to revere their world as much as, or more than my own. In one instance, a mother bear and her two baby cubs walked onto my practice, then sat down about 20 feet away and just watched. When another man appeared on the trail, the bears left, but once he had gone, they returned to join my space for another hour. This amazing experience happened on a regular basis, always when I was practicing yoga.

When I teach yoga, I often take my students out into nature and encourage them to continue to practice outdoors, at home, or on vacation, so they, too, can experience these benefits. Next time the weather is nice and you have the desire to do yoga, try surrendering your practice to the soothing hands of Mother Nature. Your body, mind and spirit will thank you… forever.

A word of caution: I am not talking about practicing yoga in the snow, the blazing heat of the desert, or especially not in a polluted environment. In adverse climatic conditions, with excessive noise or extreme pollution, you are better off practicing indoors with some plants in your room.

Practicing Yoga Outdoors & The Five Elements
Earth, Air, Fire, Water and Ether

My own personal determination to seek out and practice yoga was greatly inspired by my first teacher, the late Ernest Wood. When I was 13, he once said, "yoga is to become energy," and I have never forgotten that. After he passed away, I found myself practicing yoga out of books on nature's stage — in city parks, under the shade of mighty oak trees, alongside a meadow of wildflowers, or at the beach. I have since spent many hours practicing outdoors trying to create a mutual union with the five elements — channeling the energy and strength of earth, the lightness of wind, the warmth of sun, the fluidity of the river and the non-attachment of ether to model my practice. The results were amazing, and I felt naturally high for hours after every session.

In the right environment, the benefits of outdoor practice include enhanced pranic energy, a greater mind-body connection and heightened spiritual vision, a greater connection to all nature's creatures and most of all, discovering firsthand how the five elements of nature play a role in your yoga practice. Practicing yoga outdoors is a very educational and spiritual experience which is hard to describe in words, but if I had to pick one it would be "bliss."

It is a first-hand education from the best yoga master of all, "Mother Nature". In keeping with her teachings, life as we know it is all about energy and the five elements: earth, air, fire, water and ether. All things come from and return to these five elements.

Here are the lessons of each of the five elements:

Earth: The lesson of earth is to embrace strength, and be steadfast, grounded and unshaken in both yoga and daily life. Remain firm to your true convictions, even when surrounded by opposition on all sides.

Air: The lesson of air is to be light, free and easygoing, striving to enhance your vital life force with fresh oxygen. It also teaches us that we have a unique relationship with plants that should be honored, whereby we inhale oxygen and exhale carbon dioxide, and in exchange, plants inhale carbon dioxide and exhale oxygen.

Fire: Fire instructs us to radiate vibrant heat from our core, shed light onto higher consciousness and warm the souls of all who come into our presence. For a true spiritual experience, practice your Sun Salutations outdoors at sunrise or sunset, paying tribute to the life force energy of the sun as you feel the soothing touch of tranquility touching your very soul.

Water: Water's message is to be powerful yet soft, inspiring yet beautiful. To be flexible, able to take any form with ease, and a refreshing companion for all those you meet. Allow your life to reflect the qualities of softness and strength, as your life becomes as natural as the river flowing to the sea.

Ether: Ether is a word used to describe the void of deep space beyond our atmosphere, the invisible vacuum, which gravity, light and energy pass through. The lesson of ether is to know there are times when you should be unattached, unaffected and unshaken. In confrontations, for example, it is wise to let go, and you will avoid fueling a negative fire.

Respect this Earth
Feel the very essence of nature
In all things ...
As you embrace sacred awareness
Showing much gratitude
And appreciation
For life.

~ ~ ~

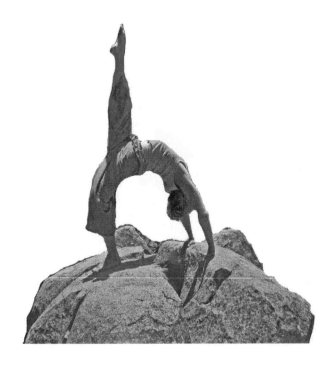

Filming the Movie
Seeking Harmony Within

"Though we travel the world over to find the beautiful, we must carry it with us,
or we will find it not." — **Ralf Waldo Emerson**

It does not matter what you do in life, how much money you make, the value of your material things, or what kind of status you represent. In the end, it is always a balancing act to maintain your own inner peace, focus and mental clarity. So, you weigh the odds, try to find the middle ground, and still keep your harmony within.

It was 1972, and I had just finished practicing my yoga under a palm tree on a Southern California beach near San Diego. The sun was setting as champagne clouds danced in the wind, floating effortlessly and free like dreams as the distant sound of waves sang a soothing, familiar melody.

I wanted to stay on my practice mat and enjoy the blissful serenity, but just down the shore crowds were gathered where a local surfing contest was underway- and I was in it. It was time to get ready for my next round "the final heat". I was sponsored at the time, with branded surf trunks and wetsuit, a company-sponsored board and even wax with the company logo.

You would think I'd be proud of these free perks, and I was, but recently they had begun to stress me out as I became increasingly weighed down by the politics of corporate surfing.

However, after my previous heats I was doing extremely well in my overall rating at the competition, favored to be a likely winner and just one step away from the finals.

So I geared up and carried my surfboard to the contestants' waiting area. After a few last minute suggestions from the team coach, I paddled out into the line-up with the five other surfers in my heat. It was a nice, sunny day with a good clean southwest swell running 4 to 6 feet amid light offshore winds. Just perfect!!!

Soon I saw a beautiful wave coming right to me. Knowing well I could impress the judges on this ride, I was already thinking of which moves would score the highest points. Yet as I started paddling into position, something strange happened. Time seemed to stop, and my mind drifted back to my yoga on the beach. I felt a longing for the non-competitive, artful practice, which always gave me a deep sense of awareness for all nature, expanding to touch every aspect of life.

As the wave approached, I saw it with the renewed sense of peace my yoga had given me. It was much larger than it looked from a distance and as the water quickly sucked up the face, I spotted a lone dolphin playing in the energy. I watched as the wave hit the shallow reef and jacked up, its beautiful blue-green lip curling upward in the golden sunlight. I spun around and began to paddle for the wave, but then something came over me, and I quickly unstrapped my leash, dove into the breaking wave and body surfed, with all my senses on high.

I was free, like the dolphin…

I was free as the sunlight and the wave

Itself…

Those few moments lasted a lifetime as I rode inside the barrel with no board. Since I was in no hurry- on nature's time- I finally reached the shore and walked up the beach, knowing full well I had lost my heat and probably my sponsor too. But I had gained a deep sense of peace, contentment and freedom.

For some time, up until that instant I had very much enjoyed competitive surfing, and the friends and sponsors who believed in me and made it all possible. But it was time for me to move on.

In one way or another many philosophers have said, "Our thoughts often create seeds and seeds grow into action." This idea was certainly true for me on that day. My subconscious had already chosen a new path and it just took one amazing yoga practice and a few subtle hints from Mother Nature to make it happen.

I officially resigned from competitive surfing and then decided to temporally detach myself from distractions to think about my next move. I even ignored my best friends who wanted to hang out. I realized I had a larger purpose than competitive surfing, so I disappeared for a few weeks, practiced yoga in remote areas, took long hikes and went soul surfing in uncrowded waves.

Then a clear vision of my dream was manifested. All I had to do was find a way to bring my idea to life. At this time in the surfing community, there were some really cool, low-budget surf movies, which inspired us surfers and the general public to play in the beauty and magic of the ocean- which also launched a fashion frenzy.

My idea was to make a beautiful film highlighting pure surfing in less traveled places. It would also weave in yoga practice in remote areas, and highlight living off the land.

It would be a documentary about searching for the perfect wave, which was not a unique idea, but the quest was just a metaphor for finding inner peace.

I wanted the movie to show that we live our whole lives and quite often cannot see the most obvious things. Yoga can instill a much deeper appreciation and gratitude for every aspect of life, both large and small. The ocean is a reflection of two kinds of energy — visible and invisible. The visible is the wave itself and the invisible is the energy pushing the wave.

Yoga creates awareness of energy and the vinyasa acts as a connecting link, uniting each asana to the next. The word vinyasa literally means 'to step or to place in a conscious manner,' and practicing this concept through yoga translates into living every aspect of life with a deep sense of awareness.

Our actions are guided by our thoughts and our thoughts then grow into our reality.

My colorful vision was to travel from one place to another, with a heightened awareness of all things, and not just surf, but become the waves, be a part of the ocean and all of life.

Yes, the movie highlighted surfing, but the message was that in daily life each separate moment is like a yoga asana, or a beautiful wave seeking only to be, and that by practicing yoga, enhanced diet and embracing deep appreciation of nature and simplicity, everyone can find "Harmony Within" without traveling anywhere.

To begin the process, I knew I had to recruit the two most wonderful souls on the planet to assist me, my little brother, David Swenson, and my best friend, Paul Dunaway. I thought it would take a great deal of time, lots of convincing and promises of fame and riches to get them on board, yet no sooner had I said "yoga and surfing" they agreed! The adventure was set.

We made a mutual alliance to be equal partners and we agreed that our message was the main motivation and much more important than trying to get rich. In the coming weeks, the three of us brainstormed ideas for possible titles of the movie and remote locations to film. We planned on what type of cameras to use, the travel logistics and getting visas. Of course we also needed some custom-made surfboards and a reliable vehicle.

It was all sounding extremely awesome except for one small detail — we added up our total combined net worth and found we had just $562.17 between us. Obviously the next order of business presented itself. We needed to get jobs to fund our yoga-surf adventure. My brother David and I decided to work at the local natural food restaurant coincidentally called "Ye Seekers Horizon." It did not pay much but had the benefit of free meals, discounted products and low stress, so we hired on. Paul, on the other hand, decided to work for his father as an assistant tugboat captain. Yes, it was a more prestigious and higher paying job, but it also carried quite a bit more stress and responsibility. So our status quickly changed from unemployed, surfer-yoga bums to respectable, actively employed citizens of society.

After work and on our time off, we met and worked out our travel plans. We decided we would film in the Caribbean, Mexico, and Central America due to their good waves, beautiful tropical flora and amazing shorelines where food grew right on the beach. We split the necessary jobs. Paul would scout around for a vehicle, I would investigate camera equipment, and David would swing some deals for new custom surf boards.

A few months later we met again and came up with an awesome idea. We decided to recruit musicians to play an original soundtrack. We all knew people who were in bands, practiced yoga and surfed too, so we bartered for free music in trade for PR and copyrights to their songs. Our musical friends jumped on board and were totally stoked to be a part of the home-grown adventure project. By chance, David knew someone who was a great artist and in time he cut a deal for him to paint a vison of our dream. This would become our movie poster.

Work, work and more work, until one day we realized we had enough capital to make our dream a reality. We set a date for March, loaded our VW van with cameras, surfboards, and yoga mats, and the adventure began.

We all agreed that Paul would bring his big German Shepherd This was mainly for security reasons, but Zariah was a cool dude too. Our journey began in South Texas, not too far from the border, so logic suggested we first travel down though Mexico, then on toward Central America.

The best thing we had going for us was that we were not on any specific schedule. We were in the moment and going with the flow of destiny.

Entering new countries is always an unpredictable adventure in itself, so we had a policy that we would pull over a few miles ahead of each border crossing and practice our yoga on a hill, in a meadow or by a river.

This way, we always confronted immigration with a relaxed energy and mental clarity. This seemed to work. We always had positive thoughts and visions of our goal, knowing that with a peaceful state of mind and good intentions the chances of success were greatly enhanced.

So all was well as we crossed the border into Mexico with no problems and we were off heading south. By the way, the roads in Mexico and Central America are not always as smooth as creamy peanut butter. They were more often goat trails through the mountains, jostling us and all of our equipment around in the van as we made our way farther and farther away from civilization.

After an eight-hour day of driving, in remote areas of Mexico, we stopped alongside a beautiful river to practice yoga and have a nice lunch. As we practiced, Zariah was swimming in the river and playing with the fish, his version of yoga.

We planned to travel across Southern Mexico the next day, and after checking our map, we decided to camp for the night so we would be fresh to make the long journey from the Gulf of Mexico to the West Coast and Pacific Ocean. All was going well. The days and weeks passed smoothly as we surfed, practiced yoga and filmed in Mexico, then moved slowly on to Central America.

One of the favorite places we discovered was a very secluded area of Costa Rica, where, to our divine pleasure, there were few people, amazing waves, and beautiful beaches lined with coconut palms, bananas and mangos, papayas, almonds, and cashews.

Weeks passed and we developed a blissful daily routine. We woke up, drank fresh coconut water and ate papaya, then paddled out into the ocean for about two hours. After surfing and filming we returned to the beach for another yoga practice under the cool shade of the palm trees. Then, it was time for a nice, healthy lunch as we relaxed. We had much gratitude for these moments in paradise. In the late afternoon, we returned for another couple hours of surfing, then bathed in the river and had an amazing dinner. We camped on a grassy area under the palm fronds, and always had peaceful dreams.

As we continued filming, after two to three weeks in one place we would travel to the next location, practice yoga, surfing, filming and living the dream. We kept going until finally we realized our money was running low. With just enough to cover gas to make the long journey back to the U.S., it was time to leave.

I think we all knew the simplicity of our daily routine during those few months would be difficult to leave behind and yet something we would remember and cherish forever.

We would also never forget the interesting locals we met along our path — farmers, fisherman and an occasional tourist.

While they were wonderful, we found our teachers and gurus in nature. The constant background sound of ocean waves, the melody of the wind through the palms, and the sweet voice of time speaking in silence.

After the trek back to the States we had mixed emotions. We were sad to give up our utopian lifestyle, but excited to finish our movie. We had to go back to work to fund the completion of our vast project. The editing was exciting and tedious, and we continued to meet with our musicians to coordinate the music to fit each separate scene.

This all took place in a simpler time. There were no personal computers, no iPhones, no digital anything. After another four or five months with lots of effort from many people who helped make the movie a reality, we had achieved our goal. We completed our low-budget, grass-roots movie, that we titled "Harmony Within," the movie pioneered a unique message, which we hoped would be a priceless gift to the public. We booked a screening tour, showing the film in college auditoriums and surf shops around the country.

In the end, we lost most of our investment, yet presented a beautiful gift to the public and gained priceless memories and a sense of accomplishment and pride in what we had done. From the beginning, financial success or failure was not our goal. We were motivated by one simple idea: "to live a natural and beautiful existence, to embrace harmony within," and at the same time sharing our vison with the public as we bring a dream to life. Success was already ours, and we hoped those who were lucky enough to see the film would appreciate what we were trying to say.

There is a sacred thread of energy which connects all living things. We are but one small piece, and those who see this will feel immense gratitude and compassion in the most simplistic moments, where peace prevails.

Sometimes this Earth spins a bit too fast. Moments, friends and surf movies- made on 8mm film- often get lost. Yet, the amazing memories they leave behind are priceless gifts which continue to light the soul in times of darkness.

~ Leave Only Wisdom ~

In the end, the greatest human who ever lived
Left only footprints in the sand...
And wisdom to expand...

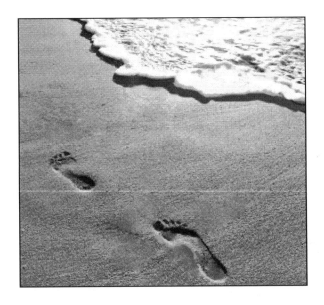

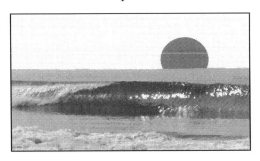

Managing Your Ego
In Yoga and Life

The ego is a part of your daily existence in each moment and every decision that arrives. You must consider if your response or action is appropriate, or if it is arising from an over-inflated ego telling you what to do like an intimidating boss. One of the best approaches in managing your ego is to first develop awareness of ego itself and then adopt an essential plan for balance. The true essence of ego can have either a positive or negative influence on your personality and greatly affect your peers, group thinking and all of society as a whole.

The definition of ego can have many different interpretations, perhaps partially because the human ego gets in the way of its own logic, much like gazing into the mirror and ignoring the things we do not want to see.

The actions and thoughts of many yoga students today reflect the shining ego controlling a driving force to achieve the perfect asana. Ironically, yoga practice in itself is designed to eliminate the ego. Therefore, we must seek a conscious approach to find clarity and balance. The ego can be your savior in times of need, or it can destroy and dismantle all things good and holy, *leading to failure and lack of integrity in yoga and life*. Looking at ego in yoga practice and beyond, I have highlighted some valuable approaches and suggestions to work with the positive side of ego, which can enhance your yoga practice. I also hope to shed light upon precautions to help avoid and overcome the negative side of your ego.

According to Freud, the mind can be divided into two main parts:

1. The *conscious* mind includes everything that we are aware of. This is the aspect of our mental processing that we can think and talk about rationally. A part of this includes our memory, which is not always part of consciousness but can be retrieved easily at any time and brought into our awareness. Freud called this ordinary memory the *preconscious.*

2. The *unconscious mind* is a reservoir of feelings, thoughts, urges, and memories that are outside of our conscious awareness. Most of the contents of the unconscious are unacceptable or unpleasant, such as feelings of pain, anxiety, or conflict. According to Freud, the unconscious continues to influence our behavior and experience, even though we are unaware of these underlying influences.

The ego arises from the conscious mind based on perception since birth and with communication from the unconscious mind.

YIN AND YANG OF MR. AND MRS. EGO

Yoga Practice and Positive Ego

On the positive side of ego, we find pride, self-esteem, and integrity, which are very beneficial and lend themselves to productivity, success, contentment, and inner peace in daily yoga practice and life. This welcome face of ego, like a good friend, is always there when we need it and helps us to be better at our yoga and our daily work — feeding us with inspiration at home and reflecting the kindness of humanity.

Yoga Practice and Negative Ego

On the negative side of ego, we find an exaggerated sense of self-importance feeding upon self-destructive energy and conceit. This side of ego is arrogant and self-infatuated, driving us to see ourselves as flawless entities. It relies on the subconscious mind to dictate irrational actions. This side of the ego becomes its own worst enemy and often takes down many innocent bystanders along its path, like a black hole in the universe.

The negative aspect of the ego tends to thrive on domination and seemingly endless control, driving forward on a quest for survival at the expense of anyone, or anything, in its path. Ego of this quality has no compassion, no genuine love or selfless generosity, and will devour sacred acts and spirituality for lunch without even blinking.

When relating directly to yoga practice, the negative side of ego can cause physical and mental injuries to ourselves and others — while causing us to adopt boxed thinking and tunnel vision.

Imagine the individual yoga student, teacher, or organization that does not want to listen to any other viewpoints, suggestions or upgrades, even if this information could help prevent injury and provide enhanced education. This would be a reflection of stubborn self-righteous pride and ego, ultimately contradicting yoga practice itself, and blocking physical and mental progress.

Needless to say, this negative side of the ego is definitely not an example of yoga integrity, philosophy or lifestyle. "Wow, dude you are harshin' my mellow!" No worries, the pleasant side of ego will arrive on wings with open arms and a warm heart to rescue you from failure.

The origins of ego extend far back to when we were young children, learning things like ownership and desire for our favorite toys or foods. As we grew, we "progressed," to striving to acquire a nice car, a trophy mate or a fancy yoga pose … "Give me that — I want it now!"

We all have stuff, yet our things should not control our lives, or define who we are. In the end, the ego-driven quest for material things offers a temporary high that leads to unhappiness, causing us to act like drug addicts looking for another fix.

In yoga practice, we should strive to extend a warm invitation to the energy of each asana, instead of trying to defeat or capture a pose for our personal possession and bragging rights.

Working Through the Ego in Yoga Practice

Yoga off the Mat

Seek yoga for the sake of yoga itself. Bathe in the art, practice and philosophy about this sacred lineage and enjoy its endless rewards both physically and mentally. Move away from doing yoga because it is cool, makes you look good, or impresses your friends. Try not to allow the title of "intermediate" or "advanced," or your teacher ranking credentials affect your integrity. Always strive to be a good example of a yoga practitioner. Yoga teachers and students are supposed to set a positive example for the rest of society, highlighting the best side of humanity.

Yoga on the Mat

Set reasonable goals and learn to enjoy the rich benefits of yoga itself rather than becoming obsessed with seeking to conquer the yoga posture, yoga routine, or style. Find the balance. There is nothing wrong with having pride in your yoga practice and looking good, or working to excel or finding support with your practice mates. But don't allow your ego to prevent you from using yoga props, or entice you to set a goal of being the best in your class or looking the most fashionable.

My Personal Accounts with Ego

From my first exposure to yoga and up until this very day, writing this book, it has always been necessary for me to keep a watchful eye on my ego, as a parent needs to watch a child to prevent him from getting in trouble. Here are a few occasions I can vividly recall when my ego was way out of balance and as result took over my words, actions and thoughts.

Ego Attacking the Asana

When I first achieved a moderate seated forward bend and had progressed far enough to be able to touch my knees, I felt an amazing sense of accomplishment, gratitude and self-esteem. Then, one thing led to another, and in time I found myself constantly hunting for new asanas so I could attack the poses, conquer them and then place them in the trophy case in my mind alongside all the other asana I had slain. In this stage of my yoga practice I was always physically injured from doing battle with my practice. My mind was not at peace.

Later on, as I matured, I made friends with my yoga postures. We loved to hang out together and explore adventures in nature. Most of all, in present times, my goal is no longer just to achieve the asana. Now I place more value on the sacred quality and art of practice itself and the feeling I have after a yoga practice, regardless of which postures I practiced or how deeply I moved.

Ego in Daily Life

There were many other times the negative side of my ego ruled my mind and actions. I suffered from excessive pride in how I looked in a photograph, or caring way too much about how I appeared in the latest fashionable yoga clothes. Another episode along my path where adverse ego took over was when I was becoming more educated about an enhanced diet. Instead of just savoring my own progress to a much healthier place physically and mentally, I placed myself on a pedestal above people I considered lower-ranking eaters. I would constantly preach to others about what they ate and I would get irritated when anyone questioned me about my diet. I thought they were not worthy of my conversation.

Today, my diet is still very strict and I am quite healthy, embracing much mental clarity, although I no longer preach to others. I choose instead to quietly set a good example. I respect the choices others make and if someone questions my diet, or tries to talk down on the way I choose to eat, I just smile, respond politely and maybe drop a few seeds of information or encouragement in a subtle manner.

What I Have Learned

From watching myself and others, I have learned we should not be so attached to the value of our material goods and riches. We should not value our net worth or status as compared to the company we keep. Humility and awareness, laced with random acts of kindness and a deep appreciation for simplicity, are the keys to the golden path. Human society would be greatly enhanced if we could only try to see the world through the eyes of others, and most of all, try to see our own true selves from a non-biased and non-egotistical perspective.

IN CONCLUSION ~

Yoga is an incredible gift. You can practice yoga without money or a car. You can practice yoga without a house or a stage. The only essential elements you really need are your motivation, a small piece of ground, and knowledge. Like a true friend, your yoga practice will always be there for you, in good times and bad.

When you lose balance, the dark side of ego can gain control of your practice and push you too far. This can cause negative repercussions both physically and mentally, so just be cool, relax and take it slow. Express gratitude for having found the sacred and priceless gift of yoga that you can carry with you throughout life.

Always remember there are some yoga postures with your name on them. These yoga postures will love you and make you look like a rock star. On the other hand, there are yoga postures that will bite you in the asana every time and make you look not so great. Just smile and practice for the sake of practice. There is no evidence to indicate that the yoga student practicing more advanced poses, or more difficult routines, is any more intelligent or spiritually enlightened than the less flexible, or less strong student.

Compassion is in love, with random acts of kindness
The ego is in love with itself...

----Doug Swenson

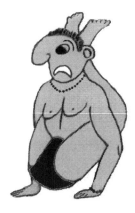

CHAPTER 15

Inspiring Vision
Of Moments in Time

After many years of practicing and teaching yoga all around the world, interlaced with surfing, meeting interesting people and embracing a very healthy diet, I have been inspired by many thoughts and opinions. These thoughts and opinions, like seeds of a tree, wanted to fill their destiny, to grow and express their true potential. From this internal energy a vision emerged and one day I wrote out a few thoughts on a piece of paper.

This urge to write began to grow, viewed through the world from a vast and often enlightened perspective, and as in all things in life, the results were partly, really good, sometimes very bad and other times down-right ugly. But I have chosen what I consider to be uplifting and educational; at the same time, this work is, at times very philosophical, and at times quite fun and interesting. These thoughts, opinions and ideas in this chapter I have chosen for you, - they are not yours to keep, yet gifts to be shared with all in the stream of life.

These Moments in Time ~ Await your Vision …

Sacred the Melody

Good Morning
Prana — keeper of this sacred practice
My effort this day
Fails to complete thee — pain & love of asana

Forty years — striving to achieve
You lend this gift to me,
Pay — I have sweat willfully
And granted by
Your destiny on moment's fate

I seek to gain — my goal of
Promised awareness & pure light —
When?
Can any Humans
Embrace semantics, the *doctor* of karma?

For so long
The seas of reason, I stormed
And if by
No greater fault — *awareness* does gift

Walk as spirit of God
Spring meadows of thought, do *await*
Yoga the divine
Best work — of nameless time

I give you now, yet
Keep it not --- for caged birds cannot fly
The future thirst …
For your soothing touch

Success listens well
    Do you …
        Listen?

Yoga Practice
    Speaks in Silence…
        Sacred the Melody

    In time …

The many

Are like fish in the ocean

Looking for *W*ater

~ ~ ~ ~

*R*esting in the woods …

Shadows ask, for life's answers

As the sun just smiles!

Knowing the one
Is treasure ~

The other, is your *K*arma

I Have Seen Beyond

I have seen beyond the practice
Walked past...
The asana and boxed rules

Tasting immense clarity
      Seeing energy as
           Fruit of the gods

Far beyond the border -

Very difficult to define
      Speaking
Without words and then hearing
      The *nectar* of this life

Where true peace is just
      Beauty of...
           Feeling aware

As moments
      Become eternity
           In the mirror of life

See everything

And you will miss nothing

~~~~

Where the few, find priceless value

Of riches- in *Simplicity*

Being in Love is Like ~

*S*wimming in an ocean

Without water

Flying into the sky
Without wings

Enjoying healthy meals
Without food

Thinking very clearly
About nothing

Staying awake at night
In case they call...

Love is the worst you can
Ever imagine

*A*nd yet ~

Love is the best thing that
Ever happened

Drink well, of this
Sweet flower nectar

As you shall be - alive...

How Do I Miss Thee

How do I miss thee? For much I concede
I look in schools, with rules, yet cannot find
I look for you, in books, speeches and deed

I miss you fully, as we strive for right
The way you touch fate, turn darkness to light
With thee, Humans future was always bright

I miss you, when countries think they need war
The way you touch minds and help spirits soar
Miss thee simplicity, passion and light

I miss your power, with grace and kind face
Miss your words of wisdom, woven as lace

Where is awareness? I have asked the sky
Man needs your compassion and mind to try

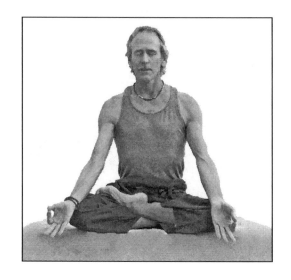

Life is Waiting

Life is more important...

Than your *ego* and money
Life is more important
Than your *status* and honey

Life is waiting - for you
Right over there
Over there
On the other side

Behind the lost thoughts
Just open your
Eyes...

And find the prize

Thought is a sunset, just waiting

For the moon
As time gazes into the reflection
Of yesterday

Chance becomes music ~

And the melody of life Unfolds...

Times Only Child

*P*racticing yoga on a lovely beach
    The air, laced passionately
As flower perfume will teach

Breezes touch softly on the mind
Easing thoughts to unwind

Palms sway gracefully
To this melody in time

Golden, the evening sun …
      Offers this lonely sea
         Light and fond memories

So forever will last

One moment
Admired by distant waves
    Of past

Gems, simplistic yet priceless
Become you …
Like eyes of the sea
Deep blue

Truly savored, by the ocean wild
Where future dreams - now believe

    In Destiny …

      *T*imes Only Child

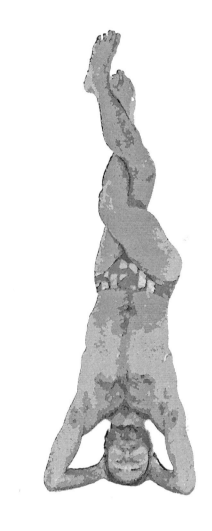

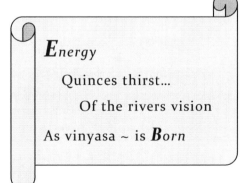

*E*nergy

    Quinces thirst...
      Of the rivers vision

As vinyasa ~ is *B*orn

CLOSING WORDS

In all aspects of your life, the most powerful weapon at your disposal is the ability to love, the most valuable tools are found within education, awareness and communication. The absence of these qualities can create poor decisions and misunderstandings, negative emotions and conflicts or even war, conversely an abundance of these qualities can prevent or even overcome these same outcomes. The solution is very simple: as a yoga student, it is your duty to uphold kindness and positive communication, strive to bridge gaps and make compromises, bend in the wind, and hold peace in your heart, as you see the world though another's eyes.

No one - individual teacher, spiritual leader, or *guru* has all the answers you need. Yet you have the answers within you. Awareness and Peace starts within, you can learn abundant, wonderful knowledge from many highly respected teachers. Yet you still must embrace all this knowledge, digesting it within your own mind, in order to create the ultimate recipe for life.

All ways are right and one way is wrong. Sunlight is nothing without the darkness and darkness needs sunlight to highlight its effects. There is a saying, "cracks within the system allow the light to shine in, and therefore you can see more clearly." Really listen when others speak, feel what is in their hearts and try to see the world within their mind, just as you would ask them, in turn, listen to you.

Much like fish in the ocean searching for water, Humans are searching the world and beyond for answers of life – many look in churches and in temples, while others look to *gurus* and philosophers, yet upon completing the cycle we will discover, for whom we have searched was our own true self. You are a part of the whole universe and the universe a part of you. It is always a great idea to seek knowledge and inspiration from others and yet in the end - true awareness, is manifested within you.

Along the journey of yoga and life,

The treasure for all mankind

Is awareness

RESOURCES

Yoga Books:

1) "Mastering Secrets of Yoga Flow" by Doug Swenson
2) "The Yoga Sutras" by: Swami Satchidananda
3) "Concentration an Approach to Meditation" by Dr. Ernest Wood
4) "The Bhagavad Gita Explained" – 1954 by Professor Ernest Wood
5) "Ashtanga the Practice" by: David Swenson
6) "Essene Gospel of Peace" by: Szekely
7) "Light on Yoga" by: B.K. S. Iyengar
8) "Hatha Yoga Pradipika" by Swami Muktibodhananda

Health Diet and Nutrition Books:

1) "Conscious Eating" - by: Gabriel Cousens M.D
2) " Miracle of Fasting" - by: Paul Bragg
3) "Become Younger" by - N.W. Walker
4) "Mucusless Diet healing System" – by: Arnold Ehret
5) "Foods That Heal " – by: Dr Benard Jensen
6) "The Hippocrates Diet" – by: Ann Wigmore
7) "The Detox Miracle Sourcebook"/ Raw Foods by: Robert S. Morse N.D.

Musical Suggestions for Meditation:

1) "Waking the Cobra" by Baird Herse (www.waking-the-cobra.com)
2) "Higher Ground" by Steven Halpern (www.stevenhalpern.com)
3) "Live on Earth" by Krishna Das (www.krishnadas.com).
4) "Medicine Power" by Oliver Shanti and friends (www.sattva.com)

Video Suggestions:

Doug Swenson has produced over 23 vidoes: See link for / **Gaia TV and U-Tube:**

https://www.gaia.com/person/doug-swenson?ch=my&filter-set=yoga&utm_campaign=1-USA-Yoga-KW-Only-Broad&utm_content=Yoga

https://www.youtube.com/watch?v=Tw_NsoXSeDk

Glossary of Yoga Asana

(Asana Glossary (English – Sanskrit)

Category # 4 Standing Poses

Category # 5 Inversions

Category # 6 Leg Stretches

Category # 7 Back Bends

Category # 8 Spinal Twist

Category # 9 Arm Balance

Category # 10 Deep Relaxation

BOOK GLOSSARY / GENERAL

GLOSSARY OF VINYASA

(Some additional vinyasa will be suggested with the asana instructions)

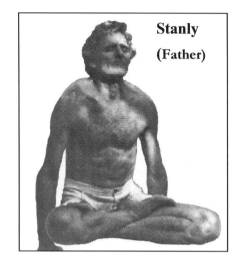

Stanly

(Father)

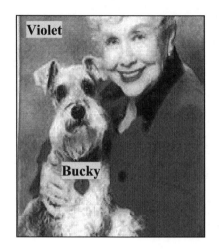

Violet

Bucky

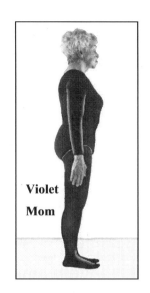

Violet
Mom

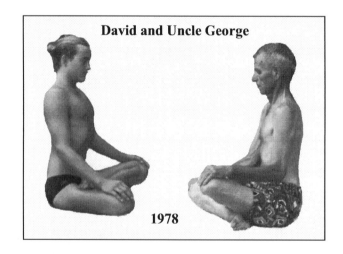

David and Uncle George

1978

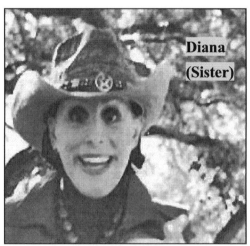

Diana

(Sister)

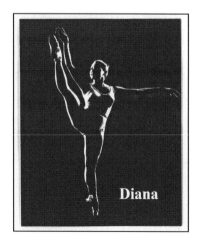

Diana

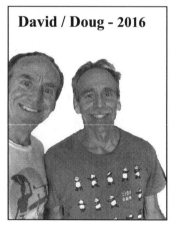

David / Doug - 2016

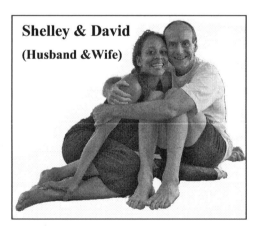

Shelley & David

(Husband & Wife)

Our Extended Family

For those who have passed before us and those still among us; we can ask the question:

Is this journey a sunrise or is it a sunset?

~ ~ ~ ~

Perception depends on where one stands in the mind's eye.
All life is a part of the same extended family;
Where many hearts of energy
Beat as one.

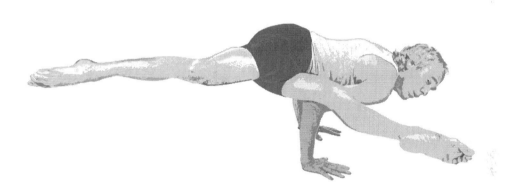

Wisdom suggests that life is a network of energy threads, mindfully woven together as a sacred blessing to all. Just as moonlight reflects upon the seas of time; we should learn to slow down and really listen, savoring the nectar in each precious moment. Our conscious effort will allow this priceless gift of life to feed souls deeper with loves gold.

When we shed light on life; awareness is born,
Thus harmony becomes our destiny
In the stream of life

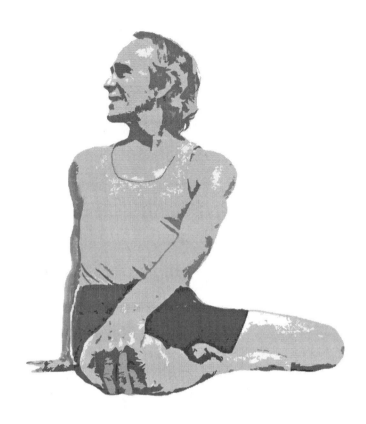

Ernest Wood wrote:

Life's fulfillment, after all, rest only

In the mind of the

Individual

Soul

Ralph Waldo Emerson wrote:

"The cordial quality of a pear or plum

Rises as gladly in a single tree

As the whole orchard resonant with bees."

Rivers of Thought ~ once ran Free

Now caged by a damn, as stagnant thoughts

Only dream of the sea

Set it free... As life must be

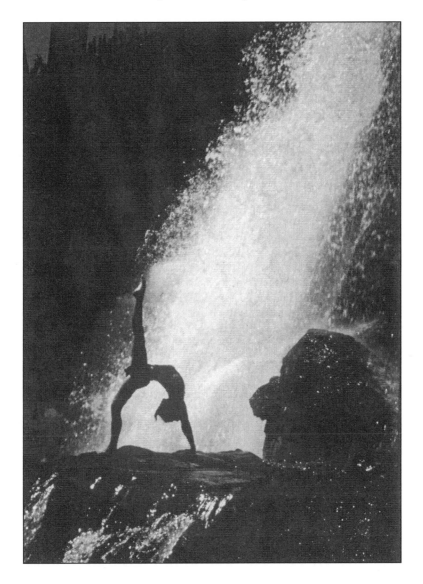

Blessing to you ~ along the sacred journey of life ☺

Namaste, Doug Swenson

ABOUT THE AUTHOR

Doug Swenson began his study of yoga in 1963, when yoga practice in most areas was considered to be weird and uncool. He has had the fortune of studying with many great teachers including: Ernest Wood, K. Pattabhi Jois, Ramanand Patel, and many others. Doug's unique approach to yoga has evolved into a holistic presentation: to include all aspects of a productive life, including enhanced nutrition, and cross-training.

Doug is a master yoga practitioner, philosopher/poet, writer and dedicated health advocate. Over the last four decades, he has incorporated influences from several different yoga systems along with his passion for healthy nutrition and conscious living to develop his own unique style of Sadhana Vinyasa Yoga. Doug is the author of several books: "Yoga Helps," "The Diet That Loves You Most," "Power Yoga for Dummies," "Mastering the Secrets of Yoga Flow" and his latest release "Pioneering Vinyasa Yoga." Doug has produced over 24 yoga videos - available on Gaia T.V. and U-tube.

The demand for his yoga teaching has led to extensive travel, around the world, teaching workshops, retreats and teacher training courses. Don't miss the opportunity to study with one of the world's top instructors. Doug's classes are always invigorating and inspirational, plus his supportive style of teaching and keen sense of humor send his student's home with a smile on their faces and softness in their hearts. Doug hosts teacher trainings at the 200, 300 and 500-hour level in Lake Tahoe, California and other locations across the U.S. and around the world.

Host Doug For: Workshops / Teacher Training Programs or Events
E-mail: dougswen002@yahoo.com / Website: www.dougswenson.net

Doug's Yoga Videos:
https://www.gaia.com/person/doug-swenson?ch=my&filter-set=yoga&utm_campaign=1-USA-Yoga-KW-Only-Broad&utm_content=Yoga

https://www.youtube.com/watch?v=Tw_NsoXSeDk